T0208918

Praise for *Health Revelations from Heaven*

"*Health Revelations from Heaven* is a bold yet loving
testimonial that elegantly explores humankind's most transcendent questions.
Through firsthand experience, Sinatra and Rosa reveal important clues
surrounding the great mystery."

—*David Perlmutter, MD, author, #1* New York Times *bestseller,* Grain Brain: The
Surprising Truth About Wheat, Carbs, and Sugar—Your Brain's Silent Killers *and* Brain
Maker: The Power of Gut Microbes to Heal and Protect Your Brain—for Life

"As one of America's foremost integrative cardiologists, Dr. Sinatra wonderfully
explains how to apply the invaluable health lessons Tommy Rosa learned on his
journey to Heaven. While not everyone has the opportunity to have an NDE, the
authors make this rare and special experience accessible—bringing Heaven and
Earth just a little bit closer."

—*Mark Hyman, MD, author, #1* New York Times *bestseller,* The Blood Sugar Solution *and*
Ultrametabolism: The Simple Plan for Automatic Weight Loss

"*Health Revelations from Heaven* is mesmerizing. For the first time, the
revelations (of Heaven) from a near-death experience have been skillfully used to
teach us how to live healthfully in our bodies right here on earth. I love this book."

—*Christiane Northrup, MD, physician, leading authority on women's health and wellness,
author of* Goddesses Never Age *and* New York Times *bestseller,* The Wisdom of Menopause

"Dr. Sinatra has always been on the leading edge in whatever he focuses his
attention on. He is one of the leaders in natural cardiology and the benefits of
grounding or earthing. In *Health Revelations from Heaven*, he provides even more
insights on how to stay healthy based on revelations gleaned from Tommy Rosa's
very special prolonged near-death experience."

—*Joe Mercola, DO, director of the Optimal Wellness Center in Chicago; founder of
Mercola.com, the world's most visited natural health site; author of* New York Times *bestseller,*
The No-Grain Diet: Conquer Carbohydrate Addiction and Stay Slim for Life

"*Health Revelations from Heaven* is equal parts informative, inspiring, and
revelatory. Told from the two fascinating perspectives of Dr. Sinatra and Tommy
Rosa, this book sheds new and much needed light on life's greatest mystery.
A powerful and brilliant work; highly recommended."

—*Nicholas Perricone, MD, FACN, CNS, board-certified clinical and research dermatologist;
author of* New York Times *bestseller,* The Wrinkle Cure: Unlock the Power of
Cosmeceuticals for Supple, Youthful Skin

"*Health Revelations from Heaven* connects you to that 'impossible to find' place through Tommy Rosa's story. We all want to know . . . what was there, what was it like, why did you come back? What are the lessons and how do we apply them to the present in order to live a better life physically, emotionally, and spiritually? Dr. Sinatra's section of the book supports that mysterious door that Tommy went through. This book really makes you want to believe and is a riveting read."

—*Suzanne Somers, actress, entrepreneur, author of multiple #1* New York Times *bestsellers, including* Sexy Forever, Knockout, *and* Ageless

"Emily Dickinson said, 'The only secret people keep is immortality.' *Health Revelations from Heaven* brings this 'secret' into the open. It's about time, because empirical evidence now shows that human consciousness extends beyond the body in space and time. The fear of total annihilation with bodily death has caused more suffering for humans than all the physical diseases combined. This book leads us beyond this grim vision to a destiny full of hope and beauty."

—*Larry Dossey, MD, physician, leader in alternative medicine and spirituality, author of* One Mind: How Our Individual Mind Is Part of a Greater Consciousness and Why It Matters *and* New York Times *bestseller,* Healing Words

"This book comes from someone who took an extraordinary trip to Heaven and came back to impart profound, life-changing lessons. Tommy juxtaposes a deeply spiritual perspective with Dr. Sinatra's practical, hands-on strategies to maintain a healthy, happy mind, body, and spirit. *Health Revelations from Heaven* will change your life, so be prepared."

—*JJ Virgin, CNS, CHFS, prominent fitness and nutrition expert, author of* New York Times *bestseller,* The Virgin Diet: Drop 7 Foods, Lose 7 Pounds, Just 7 Days

"As I read *Health Revelations from Heaven*, the tears ran down my face because I knew instinctively Tommy Rosa and Steve Sinatra were telling us the most beautiful truth about W*ho* is with us every moment and what lies beyond this life. Such honesty and clarity is rare, and I thank you for it. We live in a time when 'scientific proof' is deemed as the ultimate evidence, but Tommy, Steve, myself, and many others know there is much, much more than what can be proven with numbers. I urge you to read this book with an open and loving heart so that you, too, may receive the blessings within. Then, I urge you to carry its healing truth throughout this life so that it can be shared with all of God's children who are suffering."

—*Richard L. Becker, DO, cohost of* Your Health with Dr. Richard and Cindy Becker, *author of* Foundations for Healing: Holistic Plans for Your Return to Health and Vitality

"Every so often, you come across a book you feel compelled to read because it combines so many different aspects of life. *Health Revelations from Heaven* is one of those books. I read it, I loved it, I learned from it, and I recommend it."

—*Dannion Brinkley, near-death experiencer, author of* New York Times *bestseller,* Saved by the Light: The True Story of a Man Who Died Twice and the Revelations He Received

"In the midst of our national health disaster, to encounter a book like *Health Revelations from Heaven* is like coming upon an oasis of refreshing water and wholesome nourishment. This is an amazing collaboration between the heaven-inspired spiritual healer, Tommy Rosa, and the humane, artful, highly skilled, and down-to-earth heart doctor, Stephen Sinatra. I am certain readers who are lucky enough to read this book will find it life-changing in the best way. I heartily recommend these Revelations."

—*Robert A.F. Thurman, PhD, professor of religion at Columbia University, writer, translator, author*

"Whether you are a plumber or a heart doctor, the road less traveled always ends in the same place . . . spiritual enlightenment . . . as so evidenced in this must-read, heart-moving book. Mr. Rosa's and Dr. Sinatra's *Health Revelations from Heaven* is a beautifully orchestrated tapestry integrating mind and body, heart and soul. Don't miss out!"

—*Eva Herr, radio show host, alternative holistic counselor, author*

"Having had an NDE at age four, I know the feeling of disappointment I experienced when I didn't die. Consciousness does not die, and the experience and wisdom shared here will help you to live, learn, and accept the truth about life and so-called death."

—*Bernie Siegel, MD, physician, surgeon, author of* 365 Prescriptions for the Soul: Daily Messages of Inspiration, Hope, and Love

"For some decades, we have learned about the imperative to treat health in a holistic manner. Such an approach has included physical, emotional, social, psychological, and cultural dimensions; but now a highly regarded cardiologist includes spirituality in the mix. *Health Revelations from Heaven* takes us on the next step to an authentic holistic paradigm."

—*Nathan Katz, Bhagwan Mahavir professor of Jain studies and professor of religious studies, Florida International University*

HEALTH
REVELATIONS
from
HEAVEN

TOMMY ROSA *and* **STEPHEN SINATRA,** MD

RODALE.

RODALE
wellness

Live happy. Be healthy. Get inspired.

Sign up today to get exclusive access to our authors, exclusive bonuses,
and the most authoritative, useful, and cutting-edge information
on health, wellness, fitness, and living your life to the fullest.

**Visit us online at RodaleWellness.com
Join us at RodaleWellness.com/Join**

First published as *Health Revelations from Heaven and Earth*
in hardcover by Rodale Inc. in September 2015.
First published as *Health Revelations from Heaven* in paperback
by Rodale Inc. in August 2017.

Note: Some names and identifying details have been changed
to protect the privacy of individuals.

Book design by Christina Gaugler

Library of Congress Cataloging-in-Publication Data is on file with the publisher.

ISBN 978–1–62336–624–7 hardcover
ISBN 978–1–63565–066–2 paperback

Distributed to the trade by Macmillan

RODALE.

Follow us @RodaleBooks on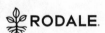

We inspire health, healing, happiness, and love in the world.
Starting with you.

146119709

This book is dedicated to all those who already see the Divine Hand in all things, including our physical and emotional healing.

And to all those seekers who are ready to take a leap of faith into understanding the mystery of the Divine Connectedness among all living beings.

CONTENTS

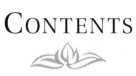

FOREWORD

by Christiane Northrup, MD

QUITE A WHILE AGO my friend and colleague Dr. Stephen Sinatra sent me a short write-up of the story of Tommy Rosa and his near death experience. And how what Tommy learned in Heaven confirmed what he did in his cardiology practice. He said that a book project was in the works. Intrigued, I kept this article nearby in a place where I could easily find it again. And I looked forward to reading the whole story. As a physician, bringing the wisdom of Heaven down to Earth was right up my alley. And I looked forward to reading the book. When the eagerly awaited manuscript for *Health Revelations from Heaven* arrived, I kept that manuscript in my bedroom—where the article had been—for months. I didn't want to lose track of it. I read every word. Even though it wasn't yet in fully edited form.

I receive countless manuscripts from individuals who are looking for endorsements. This one was different. This one—even in its infancy—found its way into my bedroom and never left—until the actual book became a reality. I can count on one hand the number of books that have affected me like this. I always know that when I can't seem to put a manuscript out of sight—where I might forget about it—I'm supposed to pay attention.

Here's what is so special about *Health Revelations from Heaven*. It's the experience of a kind-hearted regular guy—Tommy—a plumber from the Bronx—who had no prior knowledge of near death experiences. He had no preconceived notions about health or spirituality. He was brought up Catholic, and when he told his priest about his experience in Heaven, the priest didn't believe him. So the very person who should have been the most sympathetic couldn't hear it. How often good-hearted honest people like Tommy have experiences that don't fit the norm and, therefore, have had those experiences discounted by the authority figures to whom they've gone for validation. Many! And Tommy had to work through that. And the self-doubt that followed. And he writes about learning to trust himself and his experience.

Before reading Tommy and Stephen's book, I had had this notion that a near death experience would reset your life and health for good. Because you would know that there is no death. And you would also value your life enough to change any adverse habits. That's what some of the near death literature I've read had suggested.

But with Tommy, it was a different story. Despite being dead and coming back, he still found that he had lifestyle habits that he needed to overcome—specifically his weight problem and heart issues. Turns out that there is no "instant" solution for one of life's most vexing problems. Weight gain. When I had Tommy as a guest on my radio show, he said that he never did drugs or drank alcohol. But he had always loved food. He ended up in the hospital with heart problems resulting in part from his excess weight. The lesson here is that no matter who you've met in Heaven—and in Tommy's case, it was Jesus—you still have to do the work of being in a body on planet Earth! That was somehow comforting once you know that there's no getting around the work we came here to do.

Tommy writes about how, when he found out that the teacher he had in Heaven was Jesus, he had trouble accepting it. Why him? Why would a soul as advanced as Jesus want anything to do with him? This is such a universal conundrum for so many of us. Who are we to deserve such profound divine guidance and love? Tommy acknowledges that his self-esteem and self-love issues were his biggest challenges. And I know that this is true for most of us. As Dr. Bernie Siegel wrote in *Love, Medicine & Miracles*, "I've come to see that the fundamental problem most patients face is the inability to love themselves." No kidding.

One of the other astonishing parts of this book was how he and Dr. Stephen Sinatra met. Tommy knew that Dr. Sinatra, a metabolic cardiologist, could help him with his heart problem. What he didn't know was how he would meet him. It's a story that only Spirit could have organized. A perfect combination of science and intuition involving a supplement called Serrapeptase, which, quite frankly, I had never heard of until I read this book. And imagine what it was like for Dr. Sinatra to find out from Tommy that his approach to heart health and metabolic cardiology were validated by what Tommy was told in Heaven. Amazing.

At this time in history, literally millions of people are suffering from heart disease, obesity, and low self-esteem. The key to helping all of them is in this book. Not only is it full of uplifting spiritual revelations, there is also a very practical section by Dr. Stephen Sinatra that outlines a program to help heal the heart—physically.

There are no shortcuts here on Earth. And we all have to address all parts of ourselves—body, mind, and spirit. Even when we are no longer afraid of death and know that who we really are doesn't die. But while we're in a body, we have to do the work. But we don't have to do it alone. And we don't have to figure it all out on our own. In *Health Revelations from Heaven*, Tommy Rosa and Dr. Stephen Sinatra share both an incredible account of life in Heaven after death—but also a practical guidebook for how to live wholeheartedly while still on Earth in a body, including practical diet and supplement guidelines. It is so encouraging to realize that there is so much more to life than we have been led to believe. And that there are wonders in this universe beyond our ability to perceive them but which make life such a pleasure and a miracle when you know about them.

INTRODUCTION

Lessons from the Other Side

A STABBING, STEADY PAIN in my hip forced me to sit down as I exited the lecture hall. I had been speaking to a large audience in Saint Petersburg, Florida, about a vibrational healing method called grounding. It was October 2010.

I had undergone a hip replacement four months earlier, and I'd been rationalizing that the pain, though intense, must be a common side effect of that surgery, or maybe I had just been on my feet for too long that day. Either way, I had convinced myself that the pain would stop on its own.

Yet, despite my attempt at maintaining a positive attitude, the pain did not subside. In fact, as I continued to walk to the exhibit hall of alternative medicine vendors, I was in so much agony that I nearly collapsed on a bench. I looked around and rather shouted to the crowd passing me by, "Anyone have any serrapeptase?" Serrapeptase is an anti-inflammatory enzyme that can break down protein coats of microbes in the body that contribute to scar tissue, plaque, clots, and cysts.

To my surprise, a woman stepped forward and announced that she indeed had some serrapeptase. I was caught a bit off guard. Serrapeptase is something you'd normally find at a supplement vendor's booth but not something you'd expect to get from a conference attendee.

A solidly built man who was with her approached me. They introduced themselves as Tommy and Michelle Rosa and commented on how much they liked my presentation. We chatted for a few minutes. Michelle excused herself and left for her hotel room to get the serrapeptase.

I mentioned to Tommy that I was resting because of a pain in my hip.

He looked right back at me. Without skipping a beat, he said, "You have a staph infection in your right hip, and you got it recently when you had hip surgery."

I was stunned. A total stranger knew that I'd had surgery on my right hip? Impossible!

"How could you know all this just by looking at me?" I asked.

He just shrugged his shoulders and softly replied, "Spirit told me."

I was amazed that someone who was not a doctor could intuitively catch such a serious problem.

Just three weeks before the conference, I'd had surgical biopsies for lesions on my face that might be skin cancer—probably an ill-timed decision in light of my new, postoperative metallic hip. You see, *Staphylococcus aureus* is on our skin all the time. With an open incision, it can intrude into the bloodstream. And any metal in the body can be like an antenna for wandering microbes.

So staph aureus, as we medical folk call it, may localize in surgical wounds like mine. It can generate dangerous infections in the blood, bone, and skin and can be deadly serious. This microbe can stubbornly mutate and resist the very antibiotics designed to stop it. Within hospitals, staph kills tens of thousands every year.

Had it not been for this "chance" encounter with Tommy, I shudder to think what might have happened to me as the result of an untreated bacterial infection. And if you'd ever predicted that a non-medically trained attendee at one of my public lectures would be able to diagnose this in me, I wouldn't have believed you! But unlike many doctors, I'm convinced that everything happens for a reason.

It wasn't long before Michelle rejoined us, serrapeptase in hand. That's when she shared that, as she was packing to attend the conference, she had received a "message" to pack that little bottle of serrapeptase. I was instantly intrigued. Now I knew that something was going on, and I had to get to know these people better! There was some connection Tommy and I both felt in that moment. This connection would ultimately lead to a very special friendship that I cherish to this day and always will. And it would take us down a path of discovery that would be life changing for both of us—one that would completely alter the way I think about life and afterlife.

What Tommy did not immediately reveal was that several years prior, he had been in a very serious hit-and-run accident. Dead for several minutes, he was resuscitated but left in a coma for weeks. What he experienced as a result of this trauma left him a profoundly changed man who was given special insight during his "death" and became a powerful spiritual advisor in his new life after "death."

As our friendship deepened, Tommy opened up even more to me about something he had held inside for many years: that during his comatose state, he was transported by a tunnel of light to Heaven, where he met a spiritual Teacher and learned fundamentals about health and healing. I was both astonished and fascinated. I consider myself a spiritual man as well as a scientist, so it wasn't hard for me to accept Tommy's account as genuine and valid. But here I was with a man who had no medical training but could communicate with me about medicine as if he had studied it his whole life.

Tommy had what is known as a near-death experience (NDE). Throughout the documented history of man, all religions have shared one deep and common element: a belief that there is life after death. Our numerous formal accounts of man's speculation about having a soul date back to the time of the Greek philosopher Socrates (469 to 399 BC) and his student Plato. It is reported that on his deathbed, Socrates was quite calm, and he attributed that state to his belief that he was going to a better place. Plato described conversations with Greek soldiers who had "died" on the battlefield and then came back. He said that "all earthly wisdom is but a rehearsal for that great awakening, an awakening that takes place upon death."

I'm no stranger to the NDE phenomenon. For many years, I worked in emergency rooms, coronary and intensive care units, and cardiac catheterization labs where patients were suddenly brought back from the brink of death. I've heard nearly 20 NDE reports from heart attack survivors who subsequently became more intuitive, grounded, giving, and loving and less materialistic after visiting the other side. Simply put, they changed—as if their DNA (the blueprint of all life, giving instruction and function to living things) had been reshuffled. Some said they were "sent back" because it just wasn't their time. Some were "told" they were to return to this life for the sake of someone else or to accomplish something more meaningful.

For example, there's the story of Myrtle, a woman who grew up in rural Connecticut and traced her family lineage back to the Revolutionary War. She was a Daughter of the American Revolution, an accomplished violinist and horsewoman, and a person who lit up the room when she entered. She first came to me for help when she was in her early seventies.

Myrtle's doctors had not been aggressive enough in diagnosing her new and persistent symptoms. She had her husband, Harvey—a country veterinarian who really knew his stuff—drive her more than an hour to my office for an urgent visit. She'd already had a coronary artery bypass operation, so she and Harvey were quite concerned.

I examined her and knew right away that she was in trouble. I heard turbulence in the right carotid artery in her neck, and that meant blood flow to her brain was in jeopardy. She needed to be seen by a neurologist—right away. An associate in nearby Hartford agreed to examine her that same day. It turned out that the artery was so critically blocked that my colleague rushed her to immediate emergency surgery. A skillful surgeon was able to quickly restore the circulation to her brain, but Myrtle endured a cardiac arrest in the process.

Two months later, she told me the story of what happened during the operation.

While being resuscitated, she felt herself leaving her body and floating up near the ceiling, accompanied by angelic beings. Looking down, Myrtle observed the doctors and nurses frantically trying to revive her. But she realized that Harvey was not with her. After 40 happy years of marriage, Harvey was her mate, partner, business associate, and best friend. As she took in what was happening, she made a proclamation inside her mind that she thought she was verbalizing out loud:

"Oh, no! I'm not going anywhere without Harvey!"

All of a sudden, she found herself back in her body! Myrtle made the conscious decision that she was not ready. She'd worked too hard to stay alive to that point, and the journey she started just didn't feel "right" for her. So she decided to come back to her body.

In 2007, my own son, Step, weighing a mere 83 pounds and near death due to a perfect storm of metabolic, endocrine, and immune diseases, went out of body and seemingly crossed over and talked to both of his grandfathers. They gave him information that he would have had no way of knowing without that otherworldly experience. His maternal grandfather—we called him W. B.—was angry at Step, who, as a teenager, had treated his mom poorly. W. B. made Step promise "on Scout's honor" that he'd always be good to his mother.

Step asked me, "Was W. B. ever a Boy Scout troop leader? Would he use the phrase 'Scout's honor'?"

"Yes, that was him!" I said, utterly blown away, since Step had no knowledge of his grandfather's scouting background.

Step also communicated with my own dad, who said: "Tell your father [meaning me] that I'm sorry I didn't go to his last high school wrestling match."

Again, my son could not have known that my dad missed that match!

Reports of NDEs may seem like something alien to you, but I believe they are pieces of relevant evidence, chronicled throughout many centuries, that provide instructive perspective in man's search for life's overall meaning.

Once chalked up to being imagined or made up, NDEs are now being studied more seriously by scientists. Research published in the *Lancet* and the *Journal of the American Medical Association* has brought NDEs to light as events worthy of intense scientific study.

Several years ago, Tommy and I attended a Montreal conference that included lectures from international leaders in the area of NDEs. One of the speakers was Pim van Lommel, a Dutch cardiologist who interviewed 344 cardiac arrest patients and shared his findings (which were published in the *Lancet* in 2001) with us. In his presentation, van Lommel reviewed five typical elements of an NDE.

1. **An out-of-body experience.** People who have gone through a near-death experience feel that they have left their physical bodies. They can see what is happening around them or to their bodies but as though from an observer status, able to perceive their surroundings, resuscitation efforts, or surgery. Their attempts to communicate with the living people they can see and hear are unsuccessful. In these nonphysical bodies, they experience walking through walls or just "thinking" about a place and being teleported there. Notes van Lommel: "This out-of-body experience is scientifically important because doctors, nurses, and relatives can verify the reported perceptions."

2. **A holographic life review.** People recall seeing their entire life flash before them, including every act and thought, all significant and all stored away.

3. **An encounter with deceased relatives or a being of light.** People who have had NDEs often recall recognizing and meeting deceased family members in an otherworldly dimension. They may also encounter a being of light, who might be an angel or a spiritual guide. All communication is wordless, through thought transfer only.

4. **A return to the body.** Some patients are able to describe how they returned to their physical bodies after being told telepathically by the being of light or a deceased family member that "it wasn't their time yet" or that "they still had a task to fulfill."

5. **No more fear of death.** Many people who have an NDE are no longer afraid of death. This is because their afterlife experience

is so profound and real that they are sure that their spirit lives on, even if they have been declared dead by a doctor.

We were awestruck by what we heard at this conference. Tommy had experienced four out of the five NDE elements described by van Lommel!

Also, van Lommel told us that the patients repeatedly reported keen recollections of celestial experiences, even though their brains were clinically dead. He concluded that consciousness exists separately from the physical body and lives on after our earthly lives are over. In other words, death may end our physical bodies, but it isn't the end of who we are. Our spirits live on—which is exactly what Tommy was told in Heaven.

I always listen keenly to any firsthand experience of another world that people have experienced so vividly at a time when the brain supposedly was not functioning, and I've studied this intriguing subject in my own practice. My fascination had long ago caused me to ask different, more probing questions about life, death, and what happens when we die.

Are we mortal or immortal? Is something tangible actually taking place that is beyond our perception, an experience that is outside the boundaries of life as we know it and occurs when high-tech monitors no longer register any proof of life? Was I really the one bringing these people back home? Since so many people around the world have survived near death and returned from a divine experience, then where is home, really? These were the questions that occupied my mind.

My belief in NDEs had caused me considerable criticism—in large part from people who were appalled that I, a respected cardiologist and certified psychotherapist, could possibly believe in such "unscientific" phenomena.

I can't say I'm surprised by that attitude. As a physician, I know that the consensus of my profession is that we discount such experiences as dreams, interruptions in brain currents, hallucinations, and out-and-out fabrications. But because so many of my resuscitated patients recalled similar scientifically inexplicable phenomena, I was able to accept NDEs as truth. However, I had never seen a case like Tommy's, in which someone returned with so much newfound understanding of the body and its mysterious workings.

Everything Tommy told me about the fundamentals of health and healing in Heaven made real sense to me, probably because I had been practicing a similar set of theories here on Earth for decades.

You see, a long time ago, I realized that to be a truly better doctor, I needed to find ways to not just treat heart disease and other illnesses but actually prevent them in the first place. This realization was both a revelation and a no-brainer at the same time.

I'm a traditionally trained MD and longtime proponent of modern medical techniques and surgical interventions for one simple reason: They work. But I also have always known that rescuing and healing should involve more than just medical heroics. They must also be about exploring every option to keep people strong and healthy.

My approach served as a strong foundation for my interest in the relationship between behavioral and characterological traits and disease states in the body, such as the type A personality and heart disease. Someone with a type A personality is competitive, an over-achiever, a hard worker, hostile, impatient—and a person who believes that thinking is more important than feeling. And, yes, people of this "type" are more prone to heart disease; they strive to succeed without complete satisfaction or fulfillment, so much so that they deny and suppress feelings of fatigue and exhaustion, sadness, isolation, and even the physical discomforts in the chest that may be early warning signs of heart disease.

To establish health and balance within a person, the physical, mental, and emotional parts must be reintegrated—and doing so became the focus of my career as a physician and psychotherapist.

In truth, it takes commitment, emphasis, and effort to maintain your health. And it takes knowledge. You have to be aware of what is good for you and what is harmful. This can be challenging in our modern world, compared with the earliest days of our existence, when we were still hunters and gatherers and no one had to go to a gym to get exercise. Daily life was filled with running, climbing, gathering food, and escaping visible dangers like hungry predators.

Today, the dangers are less visible and obvious, but they are everywhere and increasing: We are all exposed to nutrient-stripped processed food; genetically modified organisms (GMOs) used to produce food; polluted water and air; heavy metals such as mercury, lead, and cadmium; insecticides and chemicals; cordless phones and cell phone towers; and more. Modern life and technologies are flooding the human body with toxic, unnatural elements and frequencies that cause insidious silent but deadly inflammation in the body. The list goes on and on.

With all these issues being so real, I began to emphasize many preventive measures in my practice, encouraging my patients to protect themselves from these outside influences. For example, I'd advise choosing noninflammatory, nonsugary, non-GMO organic foods such as golden organic flaxseed, extra virgin olive oil, organic kiwifruit, blueberries or blackberries, and wild migratory salmon or sardines, and adding more healthy fats, such as omega-3s, and other dietary supplements to support heart function and overall health. For those especially prone to musculoskeletal pain and weakness, I'd emphasize a similar diet, along with the avoidance of caffeine, alcohol, and food coloring and dyes, as well as toxic electric and magnetic fields, or EMFs (from cell phones, computers, and other modern-day technologies), the last of which can have a negative effect on heart rate variability (the beat-to-beat alterations in heart rate) and other aspects of health.

Most incredibly, much of this information was revealed to Tommy in Heaven!

In fact, my three most important discoveries over 40-plus years of practicing medicine were validated by Tommy's lessons in Heaven: that we can revitalize an ailing heart by natural means, that we can protect the body from illness by physically reconnecting with the Earth's energy field, and that there is a link between heartbreak and heart disease.

I was so moved by Tommy's experience that I confessed to him that I would trade all of my accomplishments for just one day in Heaven. I think Tommy knew then that I believed him with all of my heart.

What happened to Tommy is an extraordinary experience, an interaction with the divine that led to profound revelations about health and healing that are themselves true and all-encompassing. What is more amazing is how specific these revelations were—which is one of the most fascinating features of Tommy's story—and how related they were to what I had been telling my patients for years! You shall soon read about the similarities between the revelations given to Tommy and what I have written about in my previous books, including *Reversing Heart Disease, Metabolic Cardiology, The Great Cholesterol Myth, Sugar Shock, Earthing, Heartbreak and Heart Disease*, and more.

But as a preview: These revelations involved learning to let go of fear and learning to have faith. Tommy learned how we are all connected and that everything we do—good or bad—creates a ripple effect. He was made aware that everything is energy, that we determine our own physical toxicity on Earth by our actions, that we need to take care of our bodies, that our thoughts are powerful, that we have guardian angels, that life's purpose is to live through the heart, and that the only important thing in life is unconditional love. These were the lessons and messages that guided Tommy's return to life.

Tommy and I shared this material with doctors, healers, friends, and family. They were fascinated. They were moved. They were spurred to change the way they were living. They clung to this sacred information. That's when we knew that we had to bring this gift of healing knowledge to the world.

We felt that the best way to do this was through a book that could reach many people, and so we began our collaboration—one that would take us through many drafts in order to finally organize and "birth" what you are holding in your hands. We talked intensely about his experience. I shared my corroborating experiences as a cardiologist. We pored over journals and articles that matched exactly what Tommy was told in Heaven. Together we worked on presenting a linear story, beginning with what Heaven looks like and moving on to each of the revelations.

Our book addresses some fundamental yet unique questions about how to prevent health problems, heal those that arise, and stay healthy for as long as we are on Earth. It directly covers nutrition, as well as thoughts on health and healing, love, fear, the path to purpose, and other issues that deeply affect our lives.

During Tommy's stay in Heaven, eight revelations of good health were imprinted onto his psyche. They were amazingly specific and completely supported by what we know from biology, chemistry, and physics. This fact is one of the most fascinating parts of Tommy's experience; in a way, he returned from his journey with a nuanced understanding that takes medical professionals years to develop. In this book, you will read about those revelations and Tommy's journey through Heaven. After each revelation, I will show you how it is scientifically and medically validated through clinical research, as well as through my own experiences as a cardiologist. Then I'll give you recommendations on how to apply the revelation to your own life, with specific actions you can take, affirmations you can use, and simple exercises you can employ.

With the help of these divine revelations and their applications, you'll discover that you have the spiritually inspired power to heal aspects of your health and, indeed, your life. Filled with timeless knowledge and practical steps you can take right away, this is a book you'll want to refer to again and again and keep close to your heart. Read these revelations with an open mind, and know that your life will be fuller and healthier for it.

Dr. Stephen T. Sinatra

PART I

HEAVEN

CHAPTER
1

IT WAS AN ACCIDENT— OR WAS IT?

I NEVER SAW IT coming.

At around 9:00 p.m. on a chilly March evening in 1999, I was headed home after buying a loaf of bread from a neighborhood corner store a few blocks from my apartment. I had walked this route every day for 10 years. I always needed one thing or another, and I liked to walk in the evenings to unwind after 12-hour days working as a plumber. The store stayed open until 10:00 p.m. every night, so it was the perfect destination whenever I wanted some fresh air. These streets were safe, not known for criminal activity, though crazy, in-a-hurry drivers sometimes blew through stop signs or ran red lights.

I consider myself a pretty observant guy. I was always on the go in my city—the Bronx—and usually on foot. I had developed a habit of looking both ways when I crossed busy streets.

But that night was different. Maybe I was lost in my thoughts, thinking about the next day's plumbing job. To be honest, I don't remember walking at all. By the time I realized what was happening, it was already too late.

I was standing at the curb, about to cross the street, when a car with no lights on came out of nowhere. It plowed into me, and I went hurtling into the air. After I smacked down, my legs, trunk, shoulders, and head skidded on the asphalt. The friction nearly ground my skin and muscle to the bone.

I didn't see the driver. I couldn't tell you the make, model, or even the color of the car. All I can tell you is that I was 40 years old when I died.

Up until that horrible accident, I lived a pretty ordinary life. I was born into an Italian-Catholic family. We attended church regularly and observed all the traditional Catholic holidays.

I grew up in Riverdale, an Irish-Jewish neighborhood in the northwest Bronx. Riverdale is a sliver of land along the Hudson River that sits on hilly ground. Most people think of the Bronx as being a war zone with crime, drugs, and poverty—but not Riverdale. It was a tree-filled place of single-family homes, nice apartments— even mansions—with great views of the river. Riverdale provided a strong sense of community to those of us who grew up there. Today the neighborhood is filled with expensive condos and has become a very trendy place to live.

I went to Catholic school and was a pretty good student despite not studying much. After school, my friends and I hung out together. Nowadays kids don't go out; they stay glued to computer and TV screens and cell phones. It was sure different back then. With few organized activities and no hovering parents to schedule us, we took to the streets to create our own fun. It was a world of baseball, football, street hockey, and bike riding. We'd get frustrated if cars came by. I developed very muscular calves from riding my bike up and down the hills of Riverdale about an hour and a half every day.

My family lived in a two-story building, and we occupied the second floor. Next to the building was an empty lot. My friends and I used to play out there all the time. One of the trees had a swing that was a lot of fun. Riverdale was a great place for us kids.

I'd stay out until five o'clock, when my parents wanted me to come in for supper. My mom was and still is an excellent Italian cook who took great pleasure in making meals for her family. That translates into "Clean up your plate. I worked hard on this meal!" Her rich, sauce-laden dinners; the piles of bread and pasta; and our nightly desserts didn't help my waistline. I had the kind of body that used to be referred to as "husky," which is a polite way of saying "fat." Being an overweight kid made shopping for school clothes a nightmare.

My old school photos tell the story. Back then, I favored stripes paired with bold, solid colors. So you could say that as a kid, I was fat, not very stylish, and apparently somewhat color-blind.

During the summer, I'd be sent to the Catholic school camp. But I'd run away. I didn't like structure. I preferred to spend time at the swim club in my neighborhood, where there was an Olympic-size outdoor pool. My friends had the keys to open and close the place, so I got to swim after work. I swam in some local races and even won a few gold medals. The pool was a comfortable place for me. When you're overweight, water keeps you buoyant. Floating in water, you don't feel as big as you do walking on land in a giant body.

I was always an industrious kid because I liked having my own money, and I wanted to save for a car. When I was 11 years old, I got a paper route. I developed 60 to 70 regular subscribers. They liked my dependability and tipped me well. I had to get up at 5:30 a.m. to prepare my papers for delivery, so I got used to a rigorous work schedule before I was even a teenager. The papers had to be on everyone's doorstep by 7:00 a.m. I learned to work hard and fast, delivering papers by bike and sometimes on foot.

The newspaper franchise was owned by a man who was an alcoholic. He would drink away all the profits each week. Frustrated, his wife asked me to collect the money, and then lock it up for safekeeping so he couldn't get to it. I did what she asked and gave him only $50 a week. I became the gatekeeper of the profits because she trusted me.

After my paper route, I would hurry home to get ready for school. I had a long bus ride every morning, and I used that time to cram in any homework I hadn't finished the night before.

In the winter, the swim club turned into a skating rink. That's where, at age 14, I got my next job. I always loved to work, and I learned how to do every job that needed doing at the rink. I drove the power sweeper, which was great fun. I helped everyone out with their skate rentals. I sold pizza and soda at the concession stand.

The rink was the popular local hangout. Families from around the neighborhood, both parents and kids, would crowd the rink on the weekends. This was the '70s, and it was a place of carefree escapism. Back then, New York City and the surrounding boroughs were in a state of decline, with cutbacks in quality-of-life services such as the police department, the parks department, and schools. This was the era of the blackouts, too, when the power system of the city just collapsed, and millions of people were plunged into darkness. Looting erupted all over, and many buildings were burned down.

So people came to the rink to forget and have fun. I can close my eyes and it's like I'm back there. I can still hear the metal blades churning up fresh ice. I can see kids lacing up their skates. I can see girlfriends and boyfriends happily gliding hand in hand to the rich sounds of old-fashioned organ music. No one had to worry about anything. The rink was a respite—a winter wonderland in the middle of an often-chaotic city.

Through my job at the rink, I discovered that I really liked working with the public. You could say that I'm a people person: I was never too shy to strike up a conversation with a stranger, and I'm like that now. I'll talk to anybody! So it didn't take very long before I knew just about everyone who came to the rink. I enjoyed watching the good skaters practice their tricks on the ice. As for me, I was an awful skater.

My parents were diligent savers and definitely instilled in me a strong work ethic and sense of independence. They didn't believe in credit and bought only things they could afford to pay for with cash. They raised me to be the same way. I saved all my paper route money. But I knew that if I was going to buy that car someday, I needed to keep my paper route, plus work at the skating rink to speed up my savings plan.

It worked. Within weeks of getting my driver's license, I bought my dream car: a silver 1976 Mercury Cougar—a real beauty! I paid cash for it with my earnings from both jobs. It felt great to be able to do that. I was so proud of myself for being such a good saver. I've had many cars since then, but that Cougar is my favorite.

I drove it for a while, but I ended up giving the car to my father because he didn't have a vehicle of his own. My dad had ridden the bus to work every day, without complaint, for as long as I could remember. When I was able to give him that car, it made me feel really good.

My father worked hard all his life. He had served in the navy, and after World War II, he got a job as an elevator inspector. My mom was employed part-time in a clothing store. My parents rarely missed a day of work. They didn't believe in absenteeism unless you were at death's door. They set a great example for me; I went through high school with a perfect attendance record.

We didn't have all that much, but I never felt poor. We had nice Christmas holidays and took occasional vacations. Looking back, I marvel at what my parents were able to provide on so little income.

When I wasn't at school or on the job, I was helping out at home.

My parents depended upon me. I was never in trouble, and I always thought of myself as a "good boy."

When I graduated from high school, it was really time to get to work. I never went to college. I was so busy taking care of things at home that I didn't have the opportunity or time to pursue higher education. For a long time, I had it in the back of my mind that I wanted to enter the priesthood. Ultimately, I decided to go to vocational school and learn the plumbing trade. I knew several plumbers in my neighborhood, and they seemed to do okay. I was good with my hands. I liked people, so plumbing became my trade.

I enjoyed being a plumber. After a while, I went into business with a longtime friend. I would bid and plan the jobs, and I started to make a decent living. Of course, if you were bidding private jobs, there was monkey business and nepotism to deal with, but I made my fair share, and I liked my work. I was a decent plumber—an average, run-of-the-mill guy trying to do his best every day and help other people out.

Fortunately, I was able to live near my family and was proud of being able to take care of them, since everyone was getting older. When I was 23, my grandma gave me a little plot of land. I built a house for her there, from the ground up, and paid cash for it. She lived there for only three weeks before she passed away. It was sad, but I was glad to have given her a new home.

My upbringing had a positive influence on me. That neighborhood, those streets, and those jobs helped form me. It was where family was first, honesty was strength, and the core values were hard work and looking out for one another. Everything about it holds a memory, a life that's dear to me.

And then I died—and was taken to Heaven.

I DON'T REMEMBER WHAT happened on that fateful walk, and I definitely don't recall being hit. All those details were filled in for me later by others. According to those who have had similar experiences, it's not uncommon to experience amnesia regarding the events that occur just before you cross over to Heaven.

I now know that what happened to me can be classified as a near-death experience or NDE. From what I've learned over the years, NDEs have some common elements, though people who have them have their own unique experiences and encounters.

During my trip to Heaven, I was reunited with loved ones, met angels, got a glimpse of God, and learned divine teachings. I knew it was all true and not a dream or hallucination. But I felt people would think I was nuts if I told them what I saw and experienced there. Well, I did tell my mom, who told our priest, who told her I was crazy! So I kept the experience to myself for many years. I didn't even know why I was chosen to go to Heaven, because I am the most ordinary, down-to-earth guy you'd ever meet.

Now I know that God wants me to share my story with you, so that you know not only what to expect after this life is over but also how to live in the highest state of health possible, starting today. I will tell you what Heaven looked like to me: the heavenly dwellings; the angels; the flowers and trees; the mountains, lakes, and oceans; the people, babies, and animals; the schools in Heaven; and more. I'll describe my experience to the best of my ability, but anyone who has had a near-death experience will tell you that there are no words in any language that can truly capture the exquisite essence of being in Heaven.

After I tell you about Heaven, I'm going to explain the eight revelations I was given, one by one, so they can sink into your spirit. A revelation is something that might always have been evident, but few people have seen it or realized it. Sometimes it's an inspiring truth or piece of knowledge given to a person by a divine source. That's what happened to me.

With each revelation, my dear friend and coauthor, Stephen Sinatra, MD, will tell you, drawing from his expertise, why it is medically and scientifically true. Then we'll give you some action steps and exercises to show you how to apply the revelation to your life.

The essence of these revelations and Dr. Sinatra's recommendations support the fact that the body, mind, and spirit are all made of energy. Albert Einstein taught this in his quantum physics: that all things are made of vibrating energy.

If you looked at yourself under a powerful electron microscope, you'd see that you are made up of a cluster of vibrations—moving energy—in the form of atoms. And so is everything else around you—other people, animals, plants, food, and rocks. They all vibrate. So do the cells, organs, and systems in all living organisms.

A vibration, or vibe, is a distinct feeling, and it can be bad or good. You might walk through a neighborhood or city and feel a good vibe or a bad vibe. Even thoughts and emotions vibrate. A simple elevation in vibration can change depression to happiness, fear to faith, and disease to health. For example, the emotional energy of a person, place, or thing causes a vibration that can be felt by most people as positive or negative. You know this yourself. You may pick up a good or bad vibe when you are around a certain person. Our vibrations announce who we are to the world and how we might be feeling at any given time.

Vibration thus holds a special place in virtually every aspect of our lives, particularly our health—a principle that was revealed to me in Heaven and is one of the cornerstones of Dr. Sinatra's approach to healing. If you want to attract better health, for example, you must raise your vibration through your actions and choices. A higher vibration is a magnet for positive results, and a low vibration is a magnet for negative results.

Everything vibrates at a different "frequency," which is a measure of how many times something swings back and forth—for example, a playground swing, a pendulum, or your legs as you walk. These movements begin at a fixed point, then swing to another, and return to the same place at which they started. This swinging and returning back is one vibration. The more rapidly something vibrates, the higher its frequency. Frequency is measured in hertz. One hertz (or Hz for short) is one vibration per second.

Some scientists have even measured the energy frequencies of bodily organs. According to Mark Mincolla, PhD, writing in his book *Whole Health*, an American inventor and scientist named Dr. Royal Raymond Rife measured many living frequencies in the 1920s and 1930s. The heart, for example, is supposedly 67 to 70 Hz; the lungs, 58 to 65 Hz; and the brain, 4 to 30 Hz. A healthy human body has an average frequency of between 62 and 72 Hz. Rife and other early scientists felt that if the frequency drops below this range, the immune system is vulnerable to the invasion of pathogens, such as parasites, bacteria, viruses, molds, and different types of fungus. These pathogens not only affect the way the body operates but also dump harmful toxins into the bloodstream.

Many medical scientists and doctors are beginning to believe that pathogens might be wiped out safely if countered by measures that promote a higher rate of vibration. Interestingly, research on humans has already shown that exposure to frequencies of 20 to 50 Hz can help broken bones grow, mend, and become stronger, according to a 2002 report in the *Townsend Letter for Doctors and Patients*.

Mind-body interventions such as positive thinking can raise your vibration, whereas negative thinking can lower it. When you realize that your thoughts and emotions are vibrating, too, you'll appreciate the fact that you can begin to alter your health by changing what you think and how you feel. The challenge is, of course, to commit completely to the new thought patterns. Many of us are programmed from childhood to have thoughts of poor self-esteem, lack of confidence, fear, and scarcity, among others. But if you change these patterns of thoughts and feelings, you can raise your vibration and bring into your life what you truly desire—for example, better health; a happier, more positive outlook; or spiritual enlightenment.

The simplest way to accomplish this is to flood the physical, mental, emotional, and spiritual body with higher vibrational energy, which I will teach you how to do. This produces several benefits: It flushes out discordant energy, allows the body to heal itself, and reprograms your subconscious mind with a more affirmative belief system. You come to believe in yourself, that you deserve happiness and health and that virtually anything is possible for you.

How do you get to this point?

The answer is found in the eight heavenly revelations described in this book and in the medical corroboration and practices that support them. These revelations—and their real-life applications—will show you how to understand your personal vibration, elevate it, and use it to change your life and your health.

I have so much to tell you. I invite you to be my companion as I describe my journey to Heaven and back and all that I learned. Although these truths were given to me, I eventually realized that they are for all of us and can change the lives of everyone for the better. So together, we'll see what Heaven—our true home—is really like.

I hope this journey transforms you as it transformed me.

CHAPTER
2

MY JOURNEY THROUGH HEAVEN

MY MEMORY BEGINS IN a huge tunnel of brilliant white light, the brightest, purest light I've ever seen. I'm inside this tunnel, moving face first, and it envelops my entire body. The light stretches above and below me in a beautiful endless beam, without boundaries or edges. I'm being pulled deeper and deeper at a rapid speed. It blazes past me while I'm in it. I feel so much warmth and peace as I move through this light. Beautiful bright rays of colored lights, like the kind you see in time-lapse photography, streak by me. The light surrounding me in the center of the tunnel is a brilliant white, but I can also see pink and blue light at the edges of the tunnel. The tunnel is not cylindrical. It feels more like a box with no sides, but I do sense edges of light.

I feel completely at peace in a way that I've never experienced before. It is a sensation of total stillness. I instinctively know there is nothing to fear and nothing to figure out. I just somehow know to trust the process. I feel like I'm flowing within and through the light. It has a powerful, beautiful energy, and it is vibrating as if alive.

I've lost my sense of time and place. I'm surrendering to the experience, something unlike anything I've ever seen, felt, heard, touched, or known before. The scent of the air is a little familiar, a bit like the essential oils used at church. I think it's frankincense and myrrh. The smell is sweet, and the aroma comforts me. It's definitely not the smell of normal air.

After what seems like forever, I finally come to a complete stop. I find myself on my back, looking up. I feel sort of paralyzed. I can't move, but I'm not afraid, because I feel protected by this brilliant white light.

All I feel is peace.

Several minutes later, I can move again. I slowly rise to an upright position. I feel very light.

I'm in a room, and the bright light that brought me here gradually dims. As I get my bearings, I look down and realize that I can't see or feel my feet touch the ground. They're hovering just above the floor. I try moving forward a little and find myself gliding along. None of this feels weird or frightening, only natural. It's so cool!

I can see my body, my hands, my legs, and my feet. I reach over with my left hand to touch my right arm, but my hand glides right through as if my whole body is without mass. What happened to my body? I'm still me. I can think, see, hear, and feel, but I have no form, only an outline of myself. I must be in some sort of spirit form. But this doesn't scare me, because I'm wrapped in absolute peace.

The room is large with visible boundaries, as opposed to the endless light that transported me there. I'm in a strange place, for sure, but oddly, it feels familiar. The crown moldings and baseboards are trimmed with gold. The floor is white marble. Executed with great craftsmanship, not the least bit gaudy or showy, it is all very elegant and breathtaking. The room has two large mahogany chairs with massive backs and red velvet seats. On either side of the chairs are two golden candelabras, each holding 10 white candles lit from within.

Everything glows with a white but rosy tint, creating a feeling of warmth and safety. I look up and see an oddly shaped crystal chandelier decorated with unpolished, oddly shaped colored stones. They emanate light in different colors, but I can't see any power source or electricity or bulbs or wires. They are just lit from within, like the candles. The light from the chandelier reflects off the bare walls like they are giant prisms, giving off a rainbow effect. It is all just so lovely.

The room is filled with flowers, and there are so many varieties. It looks just like an English garden. I recognize white and purple lilacs and roses of every color: white, pink, yellow, red, even blue ones. The flowers outline the entire perimeter of the room. I notice that there are also large sunflowers in bloom. The combined essence of all the flowers creates a calming and peaceful effect on me. I have no fear, even though I don't know where I am.

I have no idea what has happened to me or how I got to this place. The light tunnel brought me here, but where am I? What has happened to my body? I am still me. I can think and see and hear and feel, but when I touch myself, I have no form. I am just an outline of myself. My arms and feet and torso look like me, but I can't touch myself or hold on to anything. I am totally alone in the stillness of this place. Even with all this happening to me, I feel utterly calm.

The walls are bare. There is no art or any form of decoration other than the golden inlay and hundreds of flowers. The room isn't endlessly large. It definitely has walls and many windows. The windows are clear and large and open, but there seems to be no glass. The windows start two feet above the ground and go up almost to the ceiling. They are spaced out roughly eight to ten feet apart. When I look out of the windows, all I can see is brilliant light and what looks like clouds. The clouds are very different from the clouds that I am used to seeing. They are pink and blue and a little orange, and they make the sky look like a perpetual sunset. The clouds are scattered and patchy, but I don't see any land or houses or people. I can only make out streams of colored light.

Meeting My Teacher

I'm not even wondering if I am alive or dead. It doesn't matter, because I'm so calm. I look up ahead and see the outline of a man who is filled with a light so bright that I can barely make out his features. He moves toward me. The closer he gets, the dimmer the light appears, and he gradually comes into view. I can see him more clearly, or maybe my eyes are just adjusting. I'm not sure.

This man is tall and muscular with an olive complexion. His eyes are very compelling and beautiful. They are a very soft brown and calming and seem to look right through me but in a very kind way. As I look into his eyes, there seems to be light pouring out of them, which makes his gaze very serene. He has long, thick eyelashes. His hair is shoulder length, beautifully brown and wavy, framing the kindest face I have ever seen. He isn't clean shaven, but he doesn't have a full beard, either. He has what seems like a three-week-old beard, but it is evenly grown in and doesn't look messy. He has no gray hair. His features are prominent and compelling. His face draws me in. He is smiling at me, and his smile is so warm and familiar that it makes me feel safe.

He wears an off-white robe down to his ankles that resembles something a monk would wear. His belt is knotted white silk with fringes about four inches long. He's in his bare feet, and his feet, like my own, are off the floor as he hovers about ten feet away from me. He wears no jewelry. He has a golden halo above his head, which is astonishing because it moves as he moves.

He smiles at me so warmly and with such familiarity that I feel safe in his presence—it is the kindest face I have ever seen. After a moment, he speaks to me but without moving his mouth. I hear him in my mind. This must be telepathic communication of some sort.

*Hello, Tommy.

He knows my name!

You should feel no fear, stress, or worries here. You are in a divine place.

I instinctively know to trust him. I'm safe. But more than safe—I feel a deep and perfect love flowing into me from this man. I'm humbled in his presence, and even though I have no understanding of where I am, I'm more at peace than I've ever been in my life.

Almost immediately, my "Teacher," as I see him, begins to show me my new surroundings. We move from one place to another, transported by the same tunnel of light through which I arrived.

Adjusting to this zippy form of travel, I follow my Teacher, trying to keep up with his pace. I want to be by his side. He seems almost fatherly, even though he is so young—probably in his midthirties. But he has a wisdom about him that makes him seem older.

The Beauty of Heaven

As my Teacher shows me around, I'm astonished by the luminous colors of our surroundings. There are no words in the English language—or any other language, for that matter—that can properly express what I see. But I will try to describe it anyway.

Imagine the most beautiful sunset or sunrise you have ever seen. Then imagine that the colors—the reds, the oranges, the yellows, and the lavenders—are so brilliant that they are pulsating before your eyes. It is like stepping into one of those kaleidoscopes you played

---

* *The words of the Teacher appear in italics.*

with as a child and seeing a laser light show, with the colors shifting, shining, and streaking.

But you don't just see the colors, you feel them, because you're in their midst. The feeling is one of serenity and divinity, as though you've been wrapped in a coat that takes away all the stress, brokenness, and unhappiness you've ever felt in your life.

My Teacher is eager for me to take this all in and watches me closely as I witness the magnificence around me and feel the peace within me.

As I continue to look around, I realize my senses are heightened in an incredible way. It isn't just the colors that I'm feeling, it is everything around me. The flowers! The sky! The trees! Even the air! They are vibrating and energized. It all feels like love.

I see a majestic Japanese maple tree with an umbrella of leaves extending across the magnificent sky. It's one of my very favorite trees on Earth, and here it is, standing regal and alone. I've never seen one so big. I'm connected to this tree somehow; it's alive and conscious.

As I am admiring my favorite tree, my Teacher discusses the power of trees. He tells me that trees are truly alive and each has spiritual energy that connects to the Earth's energy. The root systems of trees tie together in groups underground and are part of the Earth's natural cleansing and nourishing system. Trees radiate energy and vibrate divine unconditional love. They have their own consciousness and feelings. When you love a tree, it feels your love and radiates it back to you.

There are endless beds of flowers, including many white roses. These roses are different, though. They don't have thorns. When I ask my Teacher about this, he laughs and says no thorns are needed because the roses here do not need protection.

Everything in this garden radiates different colors: pink, red, blue, and a beautiful deep green. My Teacher sees my admiration and tells me that the grass is always green and never needs cutting. I can feel a loving energy coming from everything: plants, flowers, animals. It's nothing like Earth. The colors are alive, too.

I sense a new kind of love flowing from me. It's free of judgment, without boundaries or bad thoughts. It's all encompassing, and I feel complete.

I see people—men, women, and children—and the occasional dog and cat, also hovering as they move about. Even wild animals like tigers and lions move among the people, who stop to pet them— something that would be considered downright dangerous on Earth. I can feel that the animals are filled with as much love and peace as everything and everyone else. There are animals of every species imaginable—elephants, zebras, foxes, giraffes, and panthers.

And then something appears that sends me into utter shock and disbelief: unicorns. Have I wandered into some land of make-believe? Now I am very confused as to where I am. I honestly can't believe what I am seeing.

Until now, I thought that unicorns existed only in myths and fairy tales. But here they are! And they prance around, free. Large and majestic and as graceful as thoroughbreds, they are pure white, with the most exquisite violet eyes, and with long tapered horns spiraling out from their foreheads.

My Teacher explains that there was once a time that unicorns existed on Earth, but the planet's vibration became so low that they could no longer exist in the earthly realm. Yet because they used to populate the Earth, they have remained in the human consciousness.

Unicorns represent purity and unconditional love, and that pure love emanates from their horns, making the unicorn special and sacred. They cannot live anywhere but here, because their vibration is so high.

I can't believe it. Unicorns! They're glorious!

Much later, it would come to me that unicorns are even mentioned in the King James Bible. There's one time in Psalm 92 when the psalmist says God makes us as strong as unicorns. I'm so happily surprised by this connection. They can't be mythical, they are real!

Like all the people here, even the unicorns and other animals communicate telepathically with one and all. There seems to be only one language, and it's understood and communicated mentally. It feels, I realize with a start, like the language of love.

Guardian Angels

Everyone I see has wings, which vary in size. They are glowing, translucent, and shimmer as they move. Like fingerprints, each person's wings are just a little different—but all are astonishingly beautiful. I'm so fascinated that I can't stop staring. It's not like you see this every day! Excited by the thought, I crane my neck to see if I have wings. But to my disappointment, I'm wingless, and so is my Teacher.

With all these wings, I guess that there must be angels here, so I ask my Teacher specifically about guardian angels. Do they really exist?

> Yes, and guardian angels are a special class of angels. They occasionally appear in human form to people and animals on Earth, usually when someone is in crisis or danger or needs divine intervention and guidance. Guardian angels are devoted companions who mediate and fulfill the loving will of God toward humanity. However, they are forbidden to interfere with free will.

I know something about free will from church and sermons: It lets us make choices—to do what we want to do, to choose life or death, and to say yes or no. Free will sets humans apart from all the rest of creation. Sadly, a lot of the evil we see in the world is because of bad choices.

My Teacher knows my thoughts.

Yes, you are absolutely right. Free will is free choice, the ability to live your life as you choose. We will discuss free will in more detail later. Just know that although they do not interfere, guardian angels may illuminate a truth, reveal facts that might have been previously hidden, or help someone find lost faith. They may help a person avoid trouble before it happens. Other times, they work with you when fear has blocked your faith, and you cannot think your way out of trouble or danger. The ultimate job of a guardian angel is to inspire divinity within someone who may be overwhelmed at a particular moment in his or her life.

My Teacher explains that at birth, each of us is assigned our very own guardian angel, who may even be a deceased relative.

Each person on Earth has a guardian angel for life—a heavenly friend, grounded in genuine love rather than a sense of duty, who cares very much about your life.

I instantly wonder who my guardian angel is. Is it my Teacher, or is it someone else?

My Teacher tells me that no one knows who their guardian angel is; all I need to know is that I have one and that God assigns a guardian angel to everyone for help and protection.

Remember when you were robbed?

For a moment, I'm stunned that my Teacher knows about the scariest thing that ever happened to me.

It was Halloween, several years before, and I had gone into a part of New York City not known for its safe streets to hire a group of at-risk youths to help with small jobs in my plumbing business. I did this most Fridays with no incidents, and it made me feel like I was giving back to my community. Fridays were also payroll days, so I usually had a lot of cash in my office. Some of the kids must have watched my routine, and on the day of the robbery, they followed me back to the office.

They wore Halloween masks and took me by complete surprise. I was defenseless. First, they tied me up. Then they threw me to the ground and ordered me to keep my face to the floor. They demanded to know where the cash was. I was too terrified to think clearly, but I did as they said. I just wanted them to take the money and go.

They grabbed the cash, and I thought they would leave me alone. I was wrong. One of them walked over to where I was lying and put a gun to the back of my head. I was trembling with fear as my life flashed before me. I braced as I heard him cock the gun. Then he pulled the trigger. And nothing! Nothing! No bullet! No sound of gunshot, just cursing and the repeated clicking of his trigger filling the air. I couldn't breathe. The fear was overwhelming. Frustrated, he pulled the trigger four more times before giving up and running out the door with his accomplices. It was astonishing—his gun must have jammed. Could that have been my first experience with a guardian angel? Was a guardian angel actually there to protect me?

I know how frightened you were, my son. They did try to take your life, but it was not your time to die that day. And yes, that was your guardian angel at work.

I'm amazed to hear this. I wonder, had I survived the robbery just so I could come here at this time?

I'm jolted out of my thoughts by the sight of someone approaching us. It's a large angel. He's nearly eight feet tall, emanating a golden light, with two very large wings. His hair is blond and his eyes are blue, but, unlike my Teacher, he has no halo. He wields a gleaming silver sword with a diamond-encrusted hilt. He looks somehow familiar to me.

My Teacher introduces him as the archangel Michael.

I remember him from my Catholic upbringing. The priests

would tell us that Archangel Michael was a protector of humanity. There were breathtaking, almost lifelike statues of him adorning my Catholic school and church. His face was sculpted in a way that was soft and almost feminine.

But I can tell you with certainty that those images don't begin to capture his magnificence and the powerful energy of peace he exudes.

Archangel Michael. . . . It doesn't get any better than this!

The archangel Michael is the most powerful angel in Heaven. He works with the power of God's holy love and light to vanquish the dark, demonic forces that exist to separate humans from their Creator.

Although the archangel Michael is known as a slayer of demons, he does much more than that in service to God and to all beings. He is dedicated to helping humankind, individually and collectively.

The archangel Michael can be in many places at once so that he can help many people at the same time. If you need his help, all you have to do is to call out to him. If you say his name, he will come to assist you. You may not see him, but you will feel his powerful presence. Archangel Michael is there for everyone.

I can feel the archangel's great power and his love for me and for everything around us. I also sense the connection between Michael and my Teacher. They seem very close, almost brotherly, with a powerful love flowing between them.

Archangel Michael greets me but without words. We're together, the three of us, for a few minutes, and there is a beautiful stillness between us. And then he is gone.

Reunion with Loved Ones

I see more people at a distance. They're going in and out of houses. No one is walking; everyone is just hovering like my Teacher and I are. We move together to one of the homes, and the door swings open on its own. Shocked, I stop in my tracks. Standing before me is my father—my gentle, wonderful dad, who died of bone cancer seven years earlier. I had missed him so much since he left us. Seeing my father now in front of me fills me with absolute joy.

After we embrace, he beams at me. He looks healthier, stronger, and younger than before. There's no trace of the cancer that ate away at his bones and made him weak, listless, and a shell of his former self. As we hug, we communicate, telling each other again and again how much we miss each other. Seeing my dad there, looking so young and happy and alive, makes all the pain of losing him fade away.

In life, he was a shy man lacking in confidence who kept to himself. Now, here, he's so much more: peaceful, calm, and happy. The energy that radiates from my father feels like vibrant, unconditional love.

Another figure joins us: my grandmother, one of my most beloved relatives. She lived with us for many years, and we were very close. I was grief-stricken when she died, and I've missed her terribly over the years. I recognize her instantly, yet she looks nothing like she did during the time I knew her; here she looks like the young girl in her old photographs. How is this possible? When she died, she was almost 80 years old.

We embrace, and I feel that same love streaming from her. Energy and light glow around her head and shoulders.

I'm figuring out that everyone here has a different amount of light that radiates from their being, or I guess you could call it their spirit. Everyone I have met so far has light, which feels joyful, peaceful, and beautiful, but each person seems to radiate different amounts of light.

The power of their love is so strong. I want to ask my father and grandmother if I'm alive or have passed over to the "other side." Although my Teacher has referred to Heaven several times, I want them to confirm that this is really Heaven, but something tells me to be still and grateful for our reunion. Deep inside, I'm being told to trust what is happening and not question what I'm experiencing.

Soon my father and grandmother slip away, but not without leaving me with their energy and love.

I look to my Teacher and ask him why my father and grandma look so young.

When people, even babies and children, come here prior to age 33, they stay at the age of their death. If they are older, then they return to what they looked like at 33.

Why 33?

Thirty-three represents a master number that signifies divine promises.

I think about this statement and how many times those promises are marked for us. The 33rd time Noah's name is mentioned in the Bible is when God makes a special promise to him not to destroy the entire world again with a flood. The 33rd time Abraham's name is used in the scriptures is when Isaac, known as the child of promise, is born when Abraham is 99 years old. Thirty-three is the age at which the Son of God was crucified. Even in Buddhism, the number 33 is sacred, for it is believed that the Buddha saved mankind by assuming 33 different forms. Many other faiths have attached spiritual importance to the number 33.

Obviously, this number is significant for all, no matter if they follow the path of Abraham, Moses, Buddha, Muhammad, Krishna, or others. I sense from my Teacher that everyone is a child of God.

In Heaven, I notice that there's no segregation by religion, race, ethnicity, language, gender, social standing, or economic status.

My Teacher explains that everyone here is at different levels of divinity based on their capacity to generate and maintain Divine

Unconditional Love. Some individuals are just learning about this extraordinary love, while other individuals are fully expressed and have chosen to become love. Thus, everyone is on a different level of progression toward Divine Unconditional Love. And the larger one's wings, the further they have progressed toward that goal.

Even in Heaven there is a little healthy competitiveness!

Here, everyone works on learning how to love unconditionally. Divine Unconditional Love is the way God loves you—without judgment—and loves all the things that He has ever made. Learning how to love like God is the path to spiritual growth and enlightenment. The more like love you are, the higher your spiritual development. The goal is not to seek love but to become love.

I think about this for a few minutes. I know that on Earth, we try to find love, but how many of us try to *be* love? As for me, I've tried to be a good person, to do the right things. But am I love? Do I think this way? If I am honest, the answer is no. Maybe that's why I am here. Just as these thoughts flood into my head, my Teacher answers me.

Yes, this is why you are here. You are here to learn, so that you can become more!

As I take in this idea about becoming more, I realize this man, my Teacher, hasn't told me his name. I don't know who he is. I believe I'm in Heaven. I just saw my father who died years ago and my grandma who died years before him. I'm not walking on the ground. We are kind of flying, and everyone has wings except me and the man in front of me. This must be Heaven. Where else could we be? At the same time, I know inside that I am not supposed to ask any questions like "Who are you? Where is God? Am I alive?" I just know deep inside that I am here to listen and learn. So, instead of asking him what I really want to know, I decide to ask him more about this place and, hopefully, he will tell me later who he is and where God is.

Schools in Heaven

As I listen to my Teacher, taking in these majestic surroundings and watching the animals and people move about, I notice people going in and out of a high, multistoried building constructed from stone.

What's in this building?

This is where people come to learn sacred knowledge.

I don't understand.

Here, people continue to progress. They are given an opportunity to grow and receive knowledge regarding energy, life force, and the radiation of light and love. In the schools here, the most important lesson is about unconditional love. Each and every human being has a Divine Self. It is this Self that has the capacity to radiate unconditional love for the purpose of spiritual growth. And all self-healing is created and sustained by this love.

Much of this knowledge has been forgotten by modern man. Here, the body, mind, and spirit are studied so that what has been forgotten can be remembered and honored once more.

Wow, I'm happy to know that life here isn't just floating along on a cloud all day long.

My Teacher smiles and continues.

Everything in creation, both animate and inanimate, vibrates—from the nucleus of an atom to the molecules of your blood, your organs, light, sound, plants, animals, Earth, and the entire universe. Nothing stays still; everything moves. In the brain, these vibrations are called brain waves. They change

with your moods, thoughts, and emotions. A person's vibrations
change from minute to minute—and can run on a continuum
from low to high and anywhere in between.

The higher your vibration, the healthier you are and the
more capacity you have to grow your spirit and be of service to
those you love and to humanity at large.

I am trying to take this all in, trying to remember all the details
of what I am seeing and experiencing, so I'm burning as much as I
can into my memory as fast as I can. Maybe, if I'm learning all these
lessons, there will be a test later.

I want to be ready!

People here also learn about the chakra system, or energy
fields of the body. Each person has energy channels within the
cellular structure of the physical body. These chakras align
with specific organs in the body. The major chakras are situ-
ated in a vertical line ascending from the base of the spine to
the top of the head. For now, it is only important for you to
know that the chakras exist in each being and when people
become ill, it's because their energy fields are out of equilibrium.

Much of the information is completely new to me. I have not
studied these things before, yet it feels more like remembering than
new learning. My Teacher takes his time in slowly revealing this
information, and I am thankful. I'm fascinated but also curious as to
why he is telling me all this. Again, he knows what I'm thinking.

I want you to know and understand this sacred knowledge
because you can use it in your life, you can apply it to your
health, and you can share what you learn here with others.

This sounds to me like a huge responsibility, and I'm humbled
that he seems to think I'm up for the task. Still, what can I do? I'm

just an ordinary, blue-collar working stiff. I never went to college. I don't think of myself as supersmart, nor do I consider myself special. So, why me?

Why not you? God decides who, what, where, when, how, and why. Have faith and trust God. Put your life into His Hands. Let God be the potter; you be the clay.

As he conveys this to me, that pretty hymn "The Potter's Hand" pops into my head. I start singing, "Mold me, use me . . . I give my life to the potter's hand."

My Teacher snaps me out of my musical moment.

Before we go forward, you need to understand more about energy and how it works. You have felt the energy here. You don't need to have a college degree to understand energy. It is created by vibration. The level of a person's vibration determines his or her health.

There are many factors that lower or raise your vibration, and they're based on the physical, emotional, and spiritual choices you make. To stay healthy or to get well, you must learn how to increase your vibration. If your vibration is higher than the vibration of any opportunistic offender, such as a bacterium, virus, fungus, or other harmful microbe, then the invader cannot survive and will perish without causing damage to your body. A high vibration creates and sustains a healthy immune system.

Over time, your physicians and healers will move toward vibrational healing. They will not be the first. Many civilizations prior to your own better understood the power and promise of vibrational healing.

I take all of this in and really think about what he is saying. How could we possibly fight all the things that are making us sick? Sickness is everywhere!

My Teacher can tell what's on my mind, that I'm concerned about illnesses and how they hurt us so much.

I am teaching you these things so you can teach them yourself.

Me, a teacher? I'm a plumber. Can I do such a thing?

As I absorb this idea about me as a teacher, I realize that this man still has not told me his name. I'm not certain who he is. I have my guesses, but I know deep down that I'm here to listen and to learn, not to ask questions.

Even so, I decide to at least ask him about Heaven.

The definition of Heaven is a place where you feel Divine Unconditional Love, happiness, joy, and total peace. Is that how you feel right now? Here, with me?

Yes, I feel total peace. I feel free. I feel happy. I'm clearer, full of joy, more serene, and more connected to everything around me than ever before. I'm pretty sure I'm in Heaven.

Everything I am feeling and seeing is filling me up with awe and wonder. There are so many new ideas. I have so many questions, but my inner voice just keeps telling me to go with the flow. Before I get too lost in my own thoughts, my companion tells me in my head:

Now, close your eyes, and we will continue on our journey.

We are pulled back into the tunnel of light. We arrive at yet another building with a rainbow above it. I'm curious about the rainbow.

This is a permanent rainbow. Here, rainbows are not dependent on the weather. It never rains. On Earth, though, rain is needed. It has a cleansing effect on the Earth, washing away negativity from physical toxins and adverse energies.

What he tells me is making sense, but this insight is all so new. I have not yet wrapped my mind around it.

Now, my son, I have more to show you. It is time to learn more about that for which you are here . . . the sources of all physical, mental, and emotional well-being.

I begin to feel a sense of purpose flowing through my body. I'm ready to continue on this journey and learn truths about health, sickness, and healing—through what will turn out to be eight revelations from Heaven.

PART II

The 8 HEALTH REVELATIONS *from* HEAVEN

CHAPTER
3

THE REVELATION
of CONNECTION

AS WE MOVE THROUGHOUT Heaven, I continue to see the most glorious scenery. I guess the best way to describe it is to say it is like a highly enhanced version of Earth. There are tall, full trees; a beautiful, colorful sky; crystal clear water; and flowers filling the air with an aroma that generates a deep sense of peace. My Teacher fills me with a new stillness and a flood of unconditional love. He is preparing me for the first and most fundamental revelation—that everything, seen and unseen, is connected to everything else. What we think, do, say, and believe affects us, people in our lives, and the world around us.

There is a divine connection that exists among all things that God has ever made. This is because each of you is born from the same Divine Creational Template, making you and all living things inextricably and forever connected. There is no separation. I am connected to you; you are connected to me; and we are connected to everything and everyone else. Everything is one. You will feel this connection as we go forward.

I think about this for a moment. Aren't we distinct beings? We all seem so different from each other.

My Teacher knows I'm a little confused. He answers me with an example.

Think of snowflakes. A snowflake starts out as a simple ice crystal. As it falls from the sky through freezing air, it begins to change form, gathering water molecules and blossoming into infinitely different configurations, all because of the constantly changing conditions in the atmosphere. You will never find two snowflakes that are exactly alike. Each snowflake contributes to the beauty of the whole.

Humans are like snowflakes in that way; they come from the same source, but are all different. God creates people using the same basic combination of blood, bone, form, and DNA, making you and all living things inextricably and forever connected. Yet He endows everyone with special God-given talents and gifts, theirs to discover and use for the greater good of all. So you see, you are just like a snowflake.

His example helps me understand that I'm part of the same whole and I come from the same stuff, but I have individual gifts that I should use for good.

That is right. To further understand how everything is connected, you must first understand that everyone is born with two most precious gifts: the Divine Spark and free will.

The Divine Spark is the aspect of God that lives within each living being and binds all living things together. It is your guidepost and your link to all things divine. The Divine Spark burns brightly when you think good thoughts; live a life that reflects truth, love, honor, modesty, joy; and give service to God and others. All of these emotions and acts create an inner glow that others can perceive. It is the flow of love and warmth that makes others connect to you because it fills them with happiness to be in your presence. You are a beacon of all that is light and right and true. Through acts of charity, mercy, and faith, you continuously ignite the Divine Spark so that it illuminates your life and connects you to all things.

Conversely, acts of ego, fear, control, anger, selfishness, and faithlessness will dim the Divine Spark and thus your positive impact on others. The Divine Spark is never extinguished, but it can be dimmed by dark thoughts and acts of negativity that block out God's presence in a way that makes you feel that God is not there.

But God is always there.

I see that our goal in life is to let our Divine Spark influence us toward love, faith, giving, peace, and connection. But that this spark can go dim by bad actions, breaking our connections, and estranging ourselves from God. I feel comforted, knowing that while we may distance ourselves from God, God never distances Himself from us.

The second divine gift integral to the human experience is free will. Free will translates to the right to choose. God chose to make each individual unique, with their own special gifts. No two beings are precisely alike in that regard—like the snowflakes I talked about. Each person embodies a spiritual essence that is just theirs—specific and individual. And this spiritual essence or soul is always evolving toward its own divinity. Personal spiritual evolution, which each person directs, is based solely on one factor: choice.

Through the gift of free will, God bestows upon each of you the right to choose your own spiritual path so that you can live your life in a sacred way reflective of your truths and beliefs.

Each of you has the right to choose who you are in any given moment. Whether you choose divinely and use your life to most closely emulate God or whether you make choices that impede the growth of your soul is always up to you in every moment of your life. Who you become and how fast you get there are always up to you. You have been given everything you need to create your own unique, individualized reality. Through free will, you determine what you take from each experience in order to shape your life and guide your spiritual growth.

So you see, your choices affect you, other people, and circumstances. You must remember this, because everything is connected. You can see this in human history. There are many who stood for the right to choose, the right to decide. Wars were waged over the freedom to choose. Many were willing to lay down their lives to defend this right, this noble inalienable right.

It is helpful if people take one day of their lives and make mental notes about how they chose throughout the day. Some decisions are important and advance them spiritually, and some are just part of daily life. Once people see the many times they use the gift of free will for the good, they will feel gratitude.

But for many, the gift of free will has been abused, and this harms our divine connection. Prayers should be offered up for those who have used this gift neglectfully.

Yes, I see. Wow. We are given these gifts, and we can use them to bring wonderful things to all the situations and elements of life.

Yes. Because of the way God created the universe, each person has the potential to influence or change the course of history through the power of thought and action. Each person can create peace and tranquility within themselves and therefore

touch another life—or even influence the collective conscious-
ness of all. When one person is uplifted, others are uplifted.

Conversely, each person can also create negative, dark
thoughts and actions that negatively influence the energy of
others. When someone is negative, frustrated, defensive, or
angry, everyone they meet will feel that energy as well. This is
because thoughts, feelings, words, and actions are all forms of
energy—positive or negative—and there is a universal energy
connection among all things.

I see what he means. In my own life, positive people have
inspired me, but negative ones have discouraged me. When I'm
around people who are always complaining, criticizing, or causing
trouble, I feel down. It's the opposite with positive people: I feel
happy and peaceful.

You are called to love each other, because each life is valu-
able and cherished by God. Love is the highest form of connec-
tion. Everything that God has ever made is connected through
Divine Unconditional Love. It is this love that enables you to
love yourself and one another. Only by pulling each other
closer and opening your hearts can you ensure complete
well-being for yourself and the world in which you live. When
you increase love, caring, and connection in your life, you also
increase the health, joy, and meaning in your life—and this
can spread to others.

His words instantly bring to mind a memory, before the accident,
of the time I met a rabbi at a Marriott and we started chatting. From
the corner of my eye, I saw his child about to slip into the hotel pool,
and I grabbed him just in time to prevent him from falling in. The
rabbi was overcome with gratitude that his son had been saved and
was unharmed. In appreciation, he invited me to be a guest on his

weekly radio show, *Religion on the Line*, hosted in rotation by leaders of different faiths: a priest, a Protestant minister, and the rabbi. I was familiar with the show because I used to listen to it.

The rabbi said I could speak about anything I wished, so I talked about ways people could volunteer in the community. I created a flyer listing 10 different charities in New York City that needed volunteers. Listeners could send the radio station self-addressed stamped envelopes, and the station would send them the flyers. People responded. We got a few responses the first week, more the next week. Before long, we were getting 15 to 20 requests a week for flyers. That may not sound like a big number, but imagine the contributions those people created by connecting with others each week.

When we bring good into the lives of people we encounter—whether loved ones, casual acquaintances, or strangers we meet for the first time—our vibration increases, and that higher vibration helps raise theirs. They can then create change in the lives of those they encounter, and that love and goodness will continue to spread. I saw and experienced the power of vibrations in Heaven, and I know that this power is possible on Earth through positive connections and contributions. It's the ripple effect—a vibrational field, really. You throw a flat stone across the calm water of a pond and the ripples caused by the stone's impact continue out in ever-widening circles that touch a much larger area. And so it is with the connections we make in life.

Realizing that we are all connected—and that we are connected to God—makes me naturally want to relate to others in a kinder, more caring way. Maybe this is how we all need to approach the world we live in. It would be wonderful for the human race if we all understood and applied this revelation.

I know I can't save the whole world at once. But there are many areas in which I can do some good—or maybe a lot of good—just by caring and connecting with others. I can create ripples that might turn into huge waves. All I have to do is pick up a stone and toss it in the water. That's something any of us can do.

The Sinatra Prescription on Connection

When Tommy told me about this revelation, I was moved and inspired. I knew from my 40 years of practicing medicine that the need for connection lies at the very heart of human existence. Our ability to connect with ourselves and others is central to what makes us ill and what makes us healthy, what brings us sadness and what brings us joy, what makes us hurt and what helps us heal.

I've long known, too, that there is the connection between the healer and the patient. I feel that more than half of the healing takes place before a patient even leaves the room or takes the prescribed medicine. It is human connection—the opportunity for someone to tell their story, be listened to, and feel "seen" by another—that begins the healing process.

The most vital part of healing is that the healer fully comprehend the suffering and feelings that the patient reveals. When the patient "gets" that he or she is understood, a deeper, more profound connection is established, which in turn facilitates the healing process.

When I was a young intern on a cancer ward, I received a call at 4:00 a.m. from the nurses' station to restart an intravenous line. I had been up all night and was exhausted. Fueled by sheer adrenaline, I rushed to the patient, an elderly man who could not speak. His larynx had been removed due to throat cancer. I approached his bedside with an IV tray in hand. The man waved me off with both hands, signaling me not to proceed. He didn't want what I had to offer. I didn't fully realize it then, but all he desired was to be left alone. As I took his hand to start the IV, his profound weakness allowed me to perform the unwanted task.

Most likely, he knew that he was going to a place where IVs

didn't matter. As I worked, I noticed his knuckles and saw the letters *L-O-V-E* tattooed across the base of his fingers. The sight made me pause. I suddenly realized that here was a human being whose condition and desire were not in accord with my duty at hand. I hesitated, stopped what I'd set out to do, and sat down on the side of his bed. There was another reason for me to be there—a more important reason, it turned out.

In that moment, this gentle man rested his head on my chest. I held him and rocked him. I felt his tenderness and vulnerability. He fell asleep on me. I, too, drifted momentarily into an exhausted "nap." I came back into the awareness that in order to be a good doctor in this situation, I needed to simply sit with this man. His primary human need was love, connection, and caring, not the contents of the IV. For the first time in my training, I understood that being is much more important than doing. I experienced and learned the lesson that compassionate connection is medicine in and of itself.

Connection can even extend life. This fact has been substantiated many times by scientific research. A good example is a study done on 1,400 people with coronary artery disease. Researchers at Duke University discovered that patients with a spouse or close confidant died at one-third the rate of people who were socially alone.

However self-reliant or independent an individual may be, left alone, he or she will not endure. Whether ill or healthy or very young or very old, people need other people. It is like the Dalai Lama once said: "We can live without religion and meditation, but we cannot survive without human affection."

Globally, our connectedness is never more evident than when the world suffers a tragedy and we all mourn and pray together, regardless of how near or far we are from each other.

A good example is 9/11. Many of us recall being glued to the television and radio reports, horrified by the scenes and stories as we watched the rescue work unfold, and praying for survivors. My own connection to this event was deeply personal and frightening at the same time. I had two grown children, a son and daughter, living in New York City, close to Ground Zero. I was terrified for their safety. Thankfully, they were fine. I remember, too, after 9/11, how our human connection nationally was strengthened so enormously in spiritual and patriotic ways. People went back to church in droves and flew American flags from their homes for months. We were all connected by that singular event, both as it happened and afterward.

About 10 years later, another event—a miracle, really—connected us globally again: the 2010 rescue of 33 miners in Chile, trapped for more than two months following a shaft collapse in a gold and copper mine. The rescue operation was broadcast around the world. People everywhere prayed, captivated by the story of endurance and survival against the odds. And people everywhere cried for joy after all the miners were brought to the surface alive.

Boundaries and ideological differences melt away in those rare moments when we are all just human together. These events help us remember that we're all involved in this life together; that our connection is real and forever and precious. Just imagine what would happen if everyone around the world performed only acts of goodness and kindness. Think of the positive ripple effect this would have on our lives!

That ripple effect is produced by our own unique vibrational energy and the vibrational energy emitted by the world around us—people, relationships, nature, global events, and so forth. There is a cumulative energetic effect on our own energy patterns.

Everything in the body vibrates to its own natural rhythm. In the medical field, we refer to vibration as pulsation. The heart pulsates, red blood cells pulsate. Even our emotions and our thoughts have a vibrating or pulsating capacity. The essence of life is pulsation.

This vibrational energy can be expressed in our "aura," which is the energy field outside the body. Most people cannot see auras, but they exist around all living things. Some gifted practitioners of healing-touch therapies, such as Reiki, or the laying on of hands, claim to be able to see illnesses in the aura before they lodge themselves in the body. These healers then strive to correct the flow of energy so that disease does not enter the body.

There is simply no question that vibrational energy connects us all. We feel it every day when we meet people or encounter situations that give us good vibes or bad vibes, as Tommy mentioned earlier. We feel it in those to whom we are attracted and those from whom we pull away. We often feel that people or situations energize us or drain us. Sometimes we can even sense another person's frustration or happiness or even anger. Their emotions can enter our own energy field because we are designed energetically to absorb them. Simply stated, we are all connected—and in many, many ways.

Among the strongest proofs of human connection is that which exists between twins. I once had a patient named Jim who had a twin brother, John. During World War II, both brothers were deployed to France. Jim was safe, stationed far from enemy territory. John, on the other hand, was on the front line. But as it turned out, they were really only a heartbeat away.

One day, suddenly and without warning, Jim felt a stabbing pain that left him clutching his chest and gasping for air. He dropped the tin cup of beef broth he was holding and collapsed under an olive tree. A lifetime of thoughts flashed through his mind—the faces of loved ones and momentous events of his life.

What was happening to Jim? A heart attack? A blackout of some sort?

None of these. At the very instant Jim was struck with that stabbing pain, his brother, John, was shot with a bullet that ripped into his chest, causing white-hot pain.

Jim experienced the intense pain that was as real as the bullet wound that felled his brother.

Amazing, isn't it?

Both Jim and John survived their wartime experiences but were forever changed. They would never again take the bond of brotherhood for granted.

Reports like theirs suggest that connection can operate over long distances and is, in some individuals, highly developed. In other words, one person can sense a life-altering event that is affecting a loved one who may be very far away.

By contrast, many people are reluctant to connect or recognize and honor the connections in their lives. When I was in my early thirties, I attended a training session for psychotherapists. The instructor asked us all to take the hand of the person on either side of us. So we had to reach out—yet people were tentative, despite the fact that we were all psychotherapists in that room! We were afraid of reaching out and intermingling our personal energy with others'.

Why does this happen? I believe the answer is simple: fear of rejection. That is why so many people avoid close relationships. But people need other people. When we become isolated and lonely, the energy of depression can steal away our aliveness and connectedness to one another. It's all about energy gain versus energy drain. And when we stay disconnected, our vibration can get so low that we no longer have the energy to connect.

This fear of rejection is understandable. You've had your heart broken probably more than once, and every time, it's harder to reconnect. You'll argue with your best friend. You lose someone you love. And often, after these situations, you simply don't want to get back in the human game. It's exhausting.

But you must, or else loneliness can set in and exact a heavy toll. The loss of vital connections can injure the heart, literally. I learned this as I trained as a psychotherapist. I began to realize that there are many missing links in health and healing—namely, emotional and psychological issues such as suppressed anger. As I probed more deeply, I saw that not just anger but the loss of love—what I call

heartbreak—a lack of intimacy with other people, and emotional isolation all contribute to heart disease as strongly as smoking, diet,
inactivity, and other physical risk factors.

A number of studies have suggested a link between chronic loneliness and physical conditions such as insomnia, diabetes, heart disease, stroke, digestive upset, breathing problems, poor immunity,
migraines, and back pain. One intriguing study, published in the
January 15, 2008, issue of the *Journal of the American College of
Cardiology*, showed that chronic, ongoing anxiety significantly
increases the odds of heart attack, over and beyond what can be
explained by physical factors such as hypertension, obesity, abnormal
cholesterol, age, cigarette smoking, out-of-control blood sugar, and
other bodily cardiovascular risk factors.

What did the researchers mean by "anxiety"? They defined it by
a collection of behaviors: irrational worry and obsessive thoughts;
discomfort in interpersonal and social situations; phobias about animals, situations, or objects; and the tendency to easily experience
tension under stressful conditions. So if you experience constant ner-
vousness and social withdrawal, you may have good reason to worry
about your heart health.

Throughout life, we are constantly making connections—all
important and vital, even though they may have variable levels of
feeling. For example, a warm personal relationship may have more
depth of feeling than a connection to a job. The love for a child may
have a different meaning than the love for a spouse. All of these
examples represent connection, and they affect your core energy.
Loving, vital connections even induce the expansion and enhance
the natural ebb and flow, or rhythm, of the heart.

The loss of a vital connection can bring on heartbreak and
thereby affect the natural pulsation of the heart by causing chest
pain or erratic contractions due to the shock of the loss. Many of us
have had the painful experience of deep hurt and anguish expressing
itself in our hearts and chests.

I saw this scenario in the case of Lawrence, a 55-year-old man who came to see me. He noticed the portrait of my great-grandfather hanging in my office and told me the picture reminded him of his own father. As he spoke, Lawrence began to feel very sad and shared his life story with me. He had been born in Hungary, and after he was three years old, he never saw his father again. His father had been drafted into Hitler's army and was stationed far from home during World War II. He was captured by the Russians and died in Siberia. Throughout his entire life, Lawrence suffered a deep, unfulfilled longing for his father.

When Lawrence suffered heart disease in his late forties and needed a triple coronary bypass at age 50, he was shocked, because he had none of the traditional risk factors for heart disease. Little did he realize that his longing for his father could have damaged his heart. Over the decades, Lawrence's body had responded to his heartbreak by distorting its musculature, freezing his chest wall and making his breathing more shallow, thereby impeding circulation through his heart and lungs. The end result was heart disease. This is a form of heartbreak. Even though Lawrence had pushed aside his yearning, the physical components of this emotional wound were damaging his body.

My first and most important step was to make Lawrence aware that this heartbreak and his rigid chest were contributing factors to heart disease. He readily accepted this, which is important, because awareness is critical to healing. Next I encouraged and taught him to breathe more deeply to free up his chest and reduce its rigidity.

I also asked Lawrence to talk more with me about his sadness, thereby establishing a connection between the two of us. Once he began these simple actions, he began to heal.

I gave him permission to cry. Tears discharge toxins, so it is good for us to cry. Tears are full of stress hormones, including adrenocorticotropic hormone (ACTH), which signals the adrenals to produce cortisol, a major stress hormone that reflects the vigilance and uneasiness of uncertainty, or "waiting for the other shoe to drop." So when you cry, you release cortisol and reduce stress. A good cry literally lightens your heart by discharging sadness, anger, and other trapped emotions from your body. It's like releasing hot air from a pressure cooker. Crying often leaves us sleepy because of the loss of all that cortisol.

It is also important to express grief. What exactly is grief? I see it as the experience of loss, separation, and change—any point of ending in life: the end of a school year or a graduation, a relocation to a new city, the loss of a job, a divorce, a breakup, the empty nest, or the death of a loved one. Grief is a universal human experience; it can be painful, but it's critically important that we process our grief rather than bury it.

A study some years ago at Harvard Medical School showed a twenty-one-fold increase in heart attacks within the first 24 hours of bereavement than at other times. The researchers also noted that those at the highest cardiovascular risk were the most vulnerable to profound grief. This study confirmed earlier research that identified a heightened risk of mortality—with cardiovascular disease as the prime culprit—in the days, months, and years after the loss of a loved one. In fact, heart issues were responsible for a 20 to 53 percent increased risk in mortality after the loss of a spouse.

Unexpressed grief can become a serious risk factor for heart disease. In the grieving process, you make a connection with yourself, first and foremost. Grieving should be shared, too, not done in isolation, or you might heighten your loneliness.

There is a story told about Buddha and a mother grieving because her son had died. When the mother asks Buddha to heal her dead son, he advises her to go out into the village and gather mustard seeds from every family who has never lost a child, parent, or friend. If she finds such a household, Buddha will bring her child back to life. How many mustard seeds does she gather during her search? None—not a one. Although the mother comes back empty-handed, she returns with a deeper understanding that she is not alone in her grieving and suffering. The moral of the story is that others have had similar experiences, and we can lean on these people in our own times of need—and, in doing so, express our grief and ultimately move forward.

Through connection, we can support one another in our darkest times. We can encourage each other to know that life is more than suffering; that with hope and love, there is a way through whatever we are facing.

If you're grieving the death of someone you loved, realize, too, that there is no disconnection spiritually. In time, you'll be reunited with your loved one, as Tommy learned in Heaven. But first you have a life to live here on Earth. And that life must be lived fully.

How can you discover a sense of connection or belonging in your personal life and no longer feel separate and alone? There's no easy solution for this. It's not like you can give someone a drug or some vitamins for loneliness. I've always urged people I knew to be at risk of loneliness to get involved in something outside themselves. This could be as simple as getting a pet (for people who don't have one). A pet offers unconditional love if you're withdrawn, lonely, or grief stricken. I've sent many patients to shelters to adopt animals, and they told me afterward that it was a very heartwarming and uplifting experience. Studies show that pet owners have a fourfold better one-year survival rate after a heart attack.

If you're feeling disconnected, try giving of yourself, maybe by volunteering. You'll feel better, and so will those you help. You'll create that loving ripple effect that Tommy talked about.

Sure, I realize that sometimes it's easier to think someone else will handle a situation or take the initiative to implement positive change in the world—someone with more money, more time, more resources, more strength, more knowledge, or more ability than you. But remember, too, as Tommy's Teacher said, that we are like snowflakes, each with different gifts to create the beauty and goodness of the entire planet. Once you start sharing your gift, in cooperation with and in service to others, you'll begin to appreciate how everyone's gifts mesh perfectly for the good of the whole.

Open your heart to someone and share life experiences, emotions, and other innermost feelings. You may make a lifelong friend, as I did with Tommy. When I look back at my own childhood, it amuses me to think of how similar it was to Tommy's formative years. We were both born in New York City to Italian fathers, had paper routes as young boys, paid cash for our first cars at a young age, and were raised in the Catholic faith. Both of us even aspired to join the priesthood when we were boys.

Connect with your own family as much as possible. In 1995, I went fishing in Alaska with my brother and two sons. I discovered that hiking in the forest, fishing in the streams, watching the eagles in the sky, and sharing the habitat with bears and wolves helped me reconnect with my own body and feelings. After hours of fishing to the rhythmic motion of casting, I occasionally found myself praying to a higher power. I thanked God for giving me the opportunity to spend such precious time with my family.

Many of us feel happiness in the presence of people with whom we really wish to spend time. Interacting with loved ones creates a positive energy that springs from feelings of love. These feelings originate deep inside of us and are a tremendous source of nurturance, peace, and tranquility.

Make time to engage with the people you love, whether it's planning an activity together, talking on the phone, or even writing meaningful letters to each other. These connections will create powerful bonds that will enrich the lives of those you love.

You may also want to reconnect with the faith of your upbringing. Return to a house of worship, or quiet yourself in prayer and meditation in order to get closer to God or a higher power of your choice. Look at your own life and think about which things make you feel connected to others and to the rest of the world. Write them down and plan to do them more often. They will put you on the path to healing your body and your life.

Connection, however, should not rely so heavily on our modern technology, such as the Internet, e-mail, social media, or texting. I remember a time when I was dining at a restaurant. I noticed a father texting on his cell phone for 20 minutes while he and his little boy waited for their table. The boy kept trying to talk to his dad and engage him. But the father just ignored him and kept texting away. He was disconnected from his son's emotional needs. He didn't even look up to see that his son was crying in his aloneness, despite being in a noisy place so full of humanity. A seemingly minor drama played out in front of me, but it was an example of early childhood heart-break and abandonment—which can contribute to heart disease in adult life.

This is what is happening in our society at large. Too often, we communicate with typed words, without the resonance of the voice emanating from our heart. There is no eye-to-eye contact or human touch. It isolates us. Typing "I love you" in an e-mail or "ILU" in a text message is no substitute for saying it with your voice or in person.

God gives us opportunities all the time to honor our divine connections with each other, so actively apply this revelation to your everyday life. If you know someone else who needs a connection, the most precious thing you can do is offer your time. Share an activity, such as a meal or a movie. The one-on-one interaction is a clear signal that you care, that the person is valued. You may save someone who is hanging in the balance. In doing so, you'll expedite your own spiritual growth and raise your vibration.

As you go through your life, think about actively making as many memories as possible. Take pictures of moments with friends and family. Laugh as much as you can. Cry when you need to. Seek experiences that will bring you joy so that your cells will "dance" and vibrate with the energy of happiness, vibrancy, aliveness, and health.

When we are joyful and happy, we are less vulnerable to illness. Love like you've never been hurt, because every moment you spend lonely, unhappy, and disconnected might be a moment of health and happiness you've lost and may never get back.

There is no insignificant encounter in our passage through life. As human beings, God designed us to need and care for each other. It is part of the divine nature—that Divine Spark—that is always within us.

Applying the Revelation of
CONNECTION

Use your God-given free will to put this revelation into action in your own life. We have some steps for you—"commitment steps"—and they will help you apply this revelation and make it real for you. As you read through them, visualize yourself making a commitment to these life-changing actions. You can do them daily or weekly and, in some cases, use them in prayer or as affirmations that you can repeat to yourself and imprint on your own psyche.

- I will reach out to more people and be kinder to others with my thoughts, words, and actions. I will share a meal or a conversation. I will make a point to visit my family and enjoy experiences with them. I will give my friends and family something each time we connect. It doesn't have to be a material object. It can be a compliment, encouragement, my time, a smile, a hug, a blessing, a prayer, or any gift of attention, gratitude, caring, or love. And I will give it unconditionally, without expecting anything in return.

- I will telephone or meet in person when reaching out to someone and hope that my voice and my energy will be uplifting and healing. I realize that there's a significant difference between contact and meaningful connection, so I will not text or e-mail when I want to express love, affection, or concern. I have the power right now to produce great miracles in my life and the lives of others simply by reaching out in a positive way.

- I will give myself permission to cry or grieve. My emotions need release and should not be stuffed inside. If I need to "let things out," I will find a friend with a listening heart or seek professional or spiritual counseling if necessary. When I connect with people in difficult times, I know my soul is smiling—and so is God.

CHAPTER
4

THE REVELATION
of FAITHFULNESS

MY TEACHER SHOWS ME what the Revelation of Connection can accomplish in our lives and in the world. And he does this with so much love and divine inspiration that I accept this revelation into my heart, without doubt or question. I am now ready to go forward.

Sensing this, my Teacher tells me to close my eyes and trust him because we're going someplace new. I do so, and in a few seconds, I'm treading water in the ocean, my teacher walking beside me on the gentle waves of the sea.

What are we doing here?

We are here to perform an exercise.

Who needs to exercise? We have perfect bodies here, right?
He laughs.

No, not that kind of exercise. This is an exercise in life.

This exercise would teach me the Revelation of Faithfulness. I look into the ocean, and I can barely wrap my mind around its beauty. I love the sea, and I have swum in the Atlantic and Pacific Oceans and in the bluest waters of the Caribbean Sea. But nothing compares to the water I'm in now. Its color changes as it deepens; swaths of turquoise and indigo give way to streaks of sapphire and navy. No postcard could capture the perfection of this paradise. And everything is vibrating. My soul feels at home.

The water is so clear and crystalline that I can see all the way to the bottom. There are dolphins, turtles, and stingrays and all kinds of sea life moving below and around me.

My Teacher disappears. I'm alone again. As I search the water for him, I see in the distance several dark boats coming toward me. But the closer they get to me, the less like boats they look.

The black shapes pick up speed and come closer, causing waves to lap at my face. Oh, no—I see what they are: great white sharks with monstrous teeth, their mouths gaping open. They're heading straight for me. I go into complete and utter panic. They begin to circle me, no doubt getting ready to attack. I know I will be ripped to shreds by these terrifying creatures.

Just when I think I am done for, I hear a clear, strong, calming voice in my head. It is the voice of my Teacher.

Have no fear.

I send him back a mental message: Easy for you to say. You're not here with me. You left me here to die.

He repeats the message using a stronger tone of voice.

Have no fear.

I close my eyes and work on returning to the peace and calm I experienced only minutes earlier. I let several moments pass before opening my eyes again. To my great relief, the sharks disappear. Just like that. I let out a huge sigh of relief and slowly begin treading water again.

Just as I'm beginning to feel safe again, my Teacher materializes beside me, as if out of nowhere.

I want to teach you about the negative energy that is created through fear. You see, whatever you are afraid of in life, you will attract it to yourself. If you are afraid of getting ill, you will attract an illness to yourself. If you are afraid of being alone, you will find yourself alone for however long it takes you to relinquish that fear. If you are afraid of poverty, you will not experience abundance. If you constantly disrespect your body, you bring ravage upon your body. If you are afraid of dying, you will attract death or a deathlike experience because you will be too afraid to live.

I respond to him through my thoughts. So had I never been afraid of sharks, I wouldn't have experienced those sharks. Is that right?

Yes. The sharks would never have appeared if you had no fear of them. The moment you let go of fear, they vanished. When fear gripped you, the more afraid you became, the closer the sharks got.

So you mean whatever I'm afraid of will come to me?

Yes. That is the truth. What you fear, you will draw to yourself. Remember this, because it is sacred knowledge.

Know, too, that fear decreases your vibration and blocks people from moving forward in their lives—for example, the woman who suffers a miscarriage and is afraid to try again for fear that she will lose her baby a second time; the man who is limited in his business dealings because he is afraid to fly in airplanes; the man who is afraid to love again because his first relationship was hurtful and disappointing; or the woman who believes she will always be alone, so she doesn't create opportunities to form new relationships for fear of rejection or judgment. These fears create a lack of movement and become the shaky foundation of a fear-based life.

Fear creates a blockage to whatever it is you do want to create. So a vital step in creating anything valuable and meaningful in your life is to let go of fear.

He sees that I'm puzzled. This is a lot of new information to digest!

Fear is simply a lack of faith, because in the moments that you are succumbing to your own particular fear, you are not trusting God. How can you trust God if you are in a fearful state of mind? God is Divine Unconditional Love and Light. Where there is light, there can be no darkness. Where there is faith, there can be no fear. Faith and fear cannot coexist. If you are afraid, you are not in faith.

You are like a garden. Fear is the weed that strangles growth. Each garden must be weeded. You must pull fear out from its source. In this way, your garden will be strong and your faith will grow abundantly. And so it is!

It's a lot to think about, but that encounter with the sharks helps me understand how fear can overtake you. When I was terrified of those sharks swimming toward me, I couldn't think. All I could think about was the horror I was facing. I didn't think of God. I didn't remember to pray. I forgot everything except my fear. I couldn't think at all!

I recall how fearful I've been in different situations, and I realize now what a waste of energy this was. But can I now really let go of fear, as I have just been taught?

As I'm thinking this, my Teacher tells me that we're going to a new place where I can practice letting go of fear. All of a sudden, we're at the top of a very high peak, the highest in a vast range of mountains. I'm astonished by how majestic it all is.

What we are going to do is jump off this mountain together. I will hold your hand as we leap together.

This mountain is jutting thousands of feet into the air. Jumping off will surely kill us both. But I realize that he's serious, and we're going to do this right now.

I feel fear rising in me again as I think of us leaping. My Teacher must sense my fear mounting, because he gently takes my hand into his own. This time he doesn't disappear.

Before I know it, we're jumping and begin a rapid free fall off the mountain. Then, halfway down, I feel my hand go empty, and my Teacher disappears. It's just me now, falling a very long way down and picking up speed with every second.

I'm very scared, but my fright lasts only a few seconds before I begin to control it. I squeeze my eyes shut and breathe as best as I can. I let the fear come up, then I let it leave. It's just negative energy. I relax as I tell myself that this is all just an illusion. I realize that I'm here learning, not dying. As I continue falling, my fear begins to dissipate. It's working!

Just before crashing into the ground, my body stops abruptly. I'm vertically suspended approximately 100 feet off the ground. It's as if I am being held up by some invisible wires. My body starts to rotate downward, feet first, and I'm now hovering upright over the ground. I'm then lowered slowly and gently, and my feet eventually touch the ground.

My Teacher reappears.

You see, you let go of your fear and surrendered, so there was no devastating blow. You are learning the importance of

*conquering your fear. You are learning the power of true faith
and how it vanquishes your enemy, which is fear.*

I'm listening intently and thinking how all this time I thought
I had faith in God—but when it comes down to it, if I had faith,
why would I have been so afraid at different times in my life? I
wish I could take back some of the energy I wasted being upset or
afraid.

I find myself thinking that most people are afraid of death, and
my Teacher quickly answers my thought.

*When a person dies, the spirit is released and the physical
body ceases to function.*

What he says is an astonishing expression of hope: He's confirming what I've seen here—that we live on in spirit form!

I'm taking in so much. I guess the reason to learn anything is so
that you have a chance to do things differently. Maybe that is what
wisdom is all about. Just as I am thinking this to myself, my Teacher
places this thought into my head:

*You are correct. Wisdom is gained from experience. It is
when you are able to correct your actions and forgive yourself
and others that you can move forward away from fear and
pointless regret to take another, wiser path. This is the path to
transformation.*

Mastery over fear is such a fundamental aspect of life. Fear blocks
us. It keeps us from full involvement with the opportunities that help
us grow. Fear is only a "feeling" and not a reality. Once we acknowledge this, our thinking starts to change and the goodness of God's
universe opens up to us. We think more clearly, we make better
choices, and we draw to us situations that bring health and happiness. Faith comes in and fear goes out. Many positive things come to
us when we live in faithfulness.

The Sinatra Prescription on Faithfulness

I've been able to watch many of my patients rise above utterly hopeless situations through the power of faith. When all medical technology, pharmaceutical agents, devices, and heroic measures are exhausted, I always resort to the phrase "a hope and a prayer"—both essential aspects of faith. The case of Hope illustrates the power of faith in health and recovery.

Hope was in her late fifties and came to our hospital with intense abdominal pain. She was diagnosed with a severely inflamed bowel that required immediate surgery. Surgeons removed approximately two feet of her bowel. But following surgery, Hope deteriorated and had to undergo a second operation. At this time, doctors found an extensive amount of discolored bowel that was in jeopardy of becoming gangrenous—which meant that the tissue was dying. Because they could not remove all of her intestines, the surgeons closed her up and told me that this was a terminal and grave case.

In this seemingly hopeless situation, I offered Hope all the medical technology that was available, such as antibiotics and blood thinners. I ended my comments with optimism, and I recommended hope and prayer to Hope and her family. I didn't realize that hers was a very religious family and Hope had a strong faith in God. The family notified perhaps 100 churches all over the state of Connecticut, and thousands of people began praying for Hope.

Hope trusted that she would get well because of her strong belief and faith. She believed in getting well against all odds and intuitively "knew" she would recover. She did not waste her energy on fear, doubt, or anger but, rather, lived in the peaceful assurance afforded by her relationship with God.

A few days later, she actually began to improve. After approximately a week and a half, she was taking nutrition by mouth, and after four weeks, she walked out of the hospital. Hope had the faith that God would save her, and she survived.

What can we learn from her story? Is there a message for all of us? It was Hope's belief in a higher spiritual power that brought her into true physical healing. She trusted that she would get well, and she did get well. Hope embodied faithfulness and emanated the emotional vibrations that accompany it. She received standard medical care, but, in my opinion, it was her faithfulness and divine intervention that saved her.

WHAT EXACTLY IS FAITHFULNESS? Does it mean organized religion—that is, going to church every Sunday or to Temple on specific holidays? Is it sitting in a lotus position, completely absorbed in some meditative practice? Is it searching for a guru or belonging to a group that shares a similar belief system? Is it a positive belief in yourself, knowing that you're capable of dealing with any discouragement, handling any problem, and trusting that good will ultimately prevail, even at the most difficult junctures in life—death, disease, and danger?

Faithfulness may embrace any of these. It doesn't mean you have to believe in the conventional notion of God or go to religious services regularly. At its core, faithfulness is the confident assurance that what we hope for is going to happen.

Tommy's experience illustrates something important: that faith is the opposite of fear. Fear asks, "What bad things will happen?" Faith asks, "What great things are actually happening?"

One of the problems with fear is that it has a way of worsening situations. It feeds on itself, potentiates already high stress and anxiety levels, and attracts more of what you fear. There's an old German proverb stating that "fear makes the wolf bigger than he is," or, as Tommy might say, "Fear makes the sharks bigger than they are." In either case, this is true.

Fear can absolutely have a harmful effect on health. I recall the story of identical twin physicians, George L. Engel and Frank L. Engel. George was a pioneering psychiatrist in the field of mind-body medicine at the University of Rochester; Frank, a respected medical doctor at the Duke University School of Medicine. In 1963, at the age of 49, Frank died suddenly of a massive heart attack.

After his brother's funeral, George Engel had a physical examination. It revealed evidence of coronary heart disease, with some calcification (hardening) of his arteries. Engel then became firmly fearful that he, too, would suffer a heart attack. He wrote: "As time passed, I found myself increasingly entertaining the magical notion that if the myocardial infarction did not occur by 10 July 1964, the first anniversary of his [Frank's] death, I would survive."

True to expectation, Engel's prediction came to be. On July 9, 1964, he had a heart attack, just one day and 11 months short of the anniversary of his brother's death. Happily, Engel survived—and lived to the ripe old age of 86.

I once heard Engel speak at a conference about this experience, which he called his nemesis complex—when you fear that something tragic will happen to you. It is almost like placing a curse on your life. I was fascinated to hear Engel eloquently speak about his own fear of having a heart attack on the date of his brother's attack—and how the prophecy was fulfilled.

Many patients in my practice, particularly the young, have this incredible nemesis of fear. They, like Engel, think that they will die of a heart attack or some other disease because a sibling or parent died of a particular illness. It is difficult to say how often they are right and this actually comes true, but when I see patients with this dark belief, I counsel them that it can become a self-fulfilling prophesy if they allow themselves to buy into it. This helps them reject their own nemesis complex.

You see, the danger with the nemesis complex is that people are powerful. They can create their own disease situations and, therefore, their own destinies. The things we dwell on the most can ultimately materialize in our bodies, so we must be wary of negative expectations, because they may come true.

All living things are hardwired to feel fear as a protective response to danger and to alert us to action. But chronic, unchecked fear is a tremendously harmful emotion that can deleteriously affect the heart and the body. It makes the heart beat rapidly and forcefully. It can cause heart palpitations, constricted blood vessels, labored breathing, digestive problems, and compromised immunity. Researchers from Harvard found that anxiety and fear damage telomeres, which are the proteins at the end of our chromosomes—a situation that dramatically accelerates the aging process.

So how do you live a less fearful, more faith-filled life? There's no quick ride to faithfulness. It is a lifetime journey that requires trust, connectedness, prayer, selfless love, and a compassionate heart toward one's self and humanity.

Faith grows within our hearts, but we must devote time to nurturing this growth. Because faith cannot exist where there is fear, one way to start is to analyze the foundation of your fears. When you find yourself obsessing about something that may or may not happen in the future, use the same advice you were given as a child when crossing the street—stop, look, and listen. Bring yourself back into the present moment. Often, that which we fear never actually takes place, because our fears are not usually grounded in fact—they are grounded in feeling. We must turn off the inner voice that keeps us trapped in our fear.

Once you recognize your fears and know that they are largely baseless, learn to release them and take a leap into the unknown. As you find yourself experiencing fear, deactivate it by becoming still. Close your eyes and connect with the divine. Tell yourself: "I am not my fear; I am larger. I release it now." You'll find that the day you let go of the fears ruling your life is the day you'll actually begin to live.

I believe that we were created to live not in fear but in faith—in ourselves, in one another, and in the divine. If we stay anchored in faith, we'll no longer be terrified. We won't have the time or energy to be fearful, because we will be so filled with faith. That's because faith isn't just an attitude; it's also an action. It's about being in motion, doing things, solving problems, practicing forgiveness, seeking connections, conforming your life to your beliefs, spending time in prayer or meditation, and trusting in a divine power. Action, too, is one of the greatest ways to overcome fear, meaning that you should do what it is you fear.

Finally, have faith in the ultimate assurance: that we don't really die. Death isn't something to fear. One of the greatest gifts of my friendship with Tommy is that I am no longer afraid of death. As a doctor, I have seen death again and again. I had developed a secret fear of death, which I harbored inside myself for many years—until I met Tommy and heard his story. Tommy's experience freed me from my fear of death because it taught me that we go on; there is no real death, only the death of our bodies—our spirits live on in a place filled with beauty and divinity.

Written in the eighth century, *The Tibetan Book of the Dead*, which is a guide to be read to a dying person for instruction on overcoming the fear of death, states that the greatest single moment in this physical life is when we die and pass through a clear light into the peacefulness of the afterlife. That light is the white tunnel of light we hear so much about from people who have had near-death experiences. Tommy once told me that the purpose of that tunnel is to take us from the earthly vibration to the heavenly vibration; we need time to acclimate to Heaven's higher vibration.

This message that death is so gloriously momentous was validated for me many years ago, when I resuscitated a patient and brought him back from the brink of death. He came to my office for a follow-up appointment and promptly stated: "I want to sue you for bringing me back! Dying was the most beautiful and wonderful moment of my life."

This patient and Tommy were graced with a glimpse of Heaven. Use their experiences to help alleviate your own fear of death.

None of us should fear death. You and I—all of us—are going to a better place. Death is just a new beginning. Why be afraid if you really are going home?

Applying the Revelation of
FAITHFULNESS

Here are four commitment steps to help you apply this revelation. We recommend that you sit quietly and examine any fears that you may have, including the fear of death, and identify faith-building actions, based on our suggestions, that will help oust fear from your life and allow your faithfulness to strengthen.

- I will answer these questions: What do I fear? Rejection? Change? Failure or even success? What others think about me? The unknown? Illness? Death? I'll identify the fears that are holding me back and expose them as baseless. I'll no longer let fear keep me from pursuing my dreams or living a full life. When fear-based what-ifs come to mind, I'll tell myself, "I'll handle it." This means I'll grow from it, learn from it, and experience victory. Faith gives me the strength to make it through. I'll let go of what might happen, what should happen, or what others will think. And I'll overcome fear by doing. I will overcome my fear by verbalizing my fear aloud. For example, I will say aloud: "I don't fear being alone," or "I don't fear my body's image," or "I won't fear new relationships." "I will take a chance." "I will be committed to breaking through my fear by verbalizing it multiple times and thereby diminishing it."

- I will have trust that things happen for my ultimate good, even if I can't see the big picture. Faith is absolute trust in the divine, no matter how hopeless or how big the obstacles ahead. I recognize that faith can facilitate healing and bring back wholeness and vitality.

- I recognize that faith is a gift that grows, and I will actively grow my faith through connections of my choice, such as:

Applying the Revelation of Faithfulness (continued)

- Joining a spiritual community for the relationships, encouragement, and opportunities to take steps toward connecting to a higher power through prayer

- Meditating and finding stillness in my life

- Connecting to a higher power through prayer. Prayer can be as simple as having gratitude for your life's blessings or a conversation with your higher power. There is no specific formula. You can reach into your heart and verbalize your thoughts. You might ask for forgiveness, guidance, help, clarity, or even a divine message. But prayer should be a part of daily life even if it is for just a few minutes a day. Tommy and I always say a prayer before we meditate.

- Practicing moving meditation such as yoga or tai chi or walking while praying

- Reading spiritual texts and inspirational works

- Being in service to others through volunteering or other forms of charity

- Recognizing and being grateful for healing miracles in my life and in the lives of others

- I shall embrace the idea that there is existence after death and not be afraid of death. Those who have been drawn to the light of unending love but then are returned to Earth come back changed and more loving. I don't have to have a near-death experience to live this way. All I have to do is live more lovingly and faithfully here and now, so that when my soul is called home, I will be light in my body.

CHAPTER
5

THE REVELATION
of VITAL FORCE

As I DIGEST THE teachings about connection and faithfulness, I realize that my Teacher is building a foundation. The Revelation of Connection is experienced through relationships, including that with God. It clearly affects everyone, everywhere. I am seeing and feeling for the first time the energetic and divine threads that bind us all to each other, and to God, as one.

But in order to activate those connections, I must conquer my fears and build spiritual trust in the divine. There is a natural pattern to these revelations, and I'm beginning to see a groundwork being established for the next revelation.

My Teacher now takes me to a place that looks like a neighborhood. It has residential houses made out of brick; there are many flowers, including roses, tulips, and impatiens lining the streets. Light from above streams down in every color of the rainbow. It's magnificent. He chooses this place to tell me about the next revelation—the

Revelation of Vital Force—an inner core energy that, when strong, leads to healing, good health, and overall well-being.

He explains:

> *Vital Force is an energy that flows within us. It can also be called Life Force, General Vitality, or simply vibration. Every living thing is imbued with Vital Force at conception.*

As my Teacher continues to help me understand the importance of energy, he tells me that Vital Force and vibration are one and the same. He explains that a person's Vital Force or vibration increases or decreases throughout that person's life based on the mental, physical, emotional, and spiritual choices that are made each day. The better the choices, the higher the vibration or Vital Force and the stronger and healthier you become. A strong Vital Force makes you less prone to disease, depression, and negative thinking.

The body extracts Vital Force from nutritious food, the sun, the air, and the ground beneath our feet, as well as from positive, loving people. When we strengthen our Vital Force, our vibration increases, and the healing process is accelerated.

However, our Vital Force can be depleted by many things. Examples are toxins and negative influences, temporarily making us sick unless we give ourselves the resources to bounce back. My Teacher explains it to me this way:

> *Toxins include viruses, bacteria, heavy metals, fungi, parasites, and molds. They lower the body's vibration as they try to take over and survive. Negative emotions generated from within, like fear, lack of faith, anger, jealousy, greed, ego, self-pity, and negative thinking, also create toxins on physical and emotional levels that affect and lower your vibration.*
>
> *As the vibration of the physical body declines, the vibrations of the toxins grow stronger. Toxins feed off your Vital*

Force, and it decreases. Unhealthy cells and disease are created. Toxicity can take over a physical body if the mind, body, and spirit cannot hold and maintain a high vibration. Too much toxicity without proper cleansing allows negative energy to enter into the organs of the body.

I think to myself that this sounds like a serious problem. This must be why so many people get really sick. I can't help but wonder: How can we protect ourselves against the toxins that diminish our Vital Force? How do we properly cleanse ourselves if we've gotten off track?

An important key to staying young, vibrant, and healthy is through the mitochondria that live in every cell of the body. By nourishing the mitochondria, you fight toxic conditions of the body such as infection, disease, and many chronic illnesses. You stave off premature aging, too.

It has been a long time since I took high school biology. I don't remember much, if anything, about cellular structures, let alone "mitochondria." I'm not even sure what they are, but they must be important if my Teacher is mentioning this stuff.

I have no idea why I'm being told this. Most of this information is completely new to me. I'm just a plumber. I haven't studied these things before. It feels like they are being downloaded into my mind, almost as if I'm a computer and my brain is a computer's brain. It's not an unpleasant feeling, but I can definitely feel myself getting fuller somehow. Maybe the best way to describe the feeling is to say that I can feel myself becoming "more."

The complexity of the physical body far outshines the most advanced computer known to man. It would be like comparing the knowledge of a newborn to that of a nuclear physicist. The physical body is the most sophisticated, elegant, multifaceted system ever created. It is a complex combination of many different systems, all interconnected, all working simultaneously to sustain life. And like a modern-day computer, the body performs thousands of internal functions each second.

So, I ask my Teacher, "Can you tell me a good way to stay physically healthy when going through life?"

Yes. That is another good question. You will understand more later, but for now, let me say that the physical body was created to heal itself as long as it is given the positive resources to do so. It is truly a perfect healing machine, but it has an interdependence on physical, mental, and emotional well-being, all within your power.

I'm eager to learn more about how my body works. I am trying to grasp how one tiny part of a cell could possibly control all of life. I'm in awe about the knowledge being given to me—and humbly grateful that God designed our bodies so wonderfully that they can self-heal under the right conditions. In the past, I just took my medicine and went about my life. The human body is remarkable, if you think about it. It kills germs. It repairs cuts. It knits bones back together. It regenerates tissues. All of this is driven by our Vital Force.

When our Vital Force is kept strong, our vibration is higher, and healing is all the quicker and more complete. I want to take this revelation more seriously. It builds the foundation for health and well-being.

The Sinatra Prescription on Vital Force

After I got to know Tommy better, I really quizzed him about any medical science revealed to him by his Teacher. Did he really talk about mitochondria? It was hard for me to comprehend how incredible it was that Tommy had received all of this information.

Tommy told me that, yes, his Teacher explained all of those things. I was stunned and excited at the same time. For one thing, I knew from my medical practice that when mitochondria and ATP are supported, not only can organs, particularly the heart, be repaired, but they can also be rejuvenated.

So what Tommy heard and learned was absolutely correct. Without going into too much detail, here is what it means medically.

Mitochondria are tiny cucumber-shaped power plants in cells that generate this Vital Force, which we call ATP. It stands for adenosine triphosphate. Mitochondria are energy factories in your cells. Using the food you eat, they produce your Vital Force. This Vital Force is called chi by the Chinese, ki by the Japanese, prana by Hindus, and breath of God by Hebrews and Christians. ATP is a molecule that powers the activities of every cell. In all of these traditions, when that Vital Force is interrupted or cut off, disease occurs. But when that energy is restored, cells are revived, and the body begins to heal.

ATP is the energy of life, and our body must make it continuously or else we perish. We store enough for only 8 to 10 heartbeats. The food we eat and the air we breathe are converted to ATP, which then drives all the metabolic reactions in the body to sustain life.

In all forms of heart disease—especially congestive heart failure (CHF)—there is dysfunctional metabolism of ATP, creating a relentless deficit. CHF is literally an "energy-starved heart." When ATP levels drop, the heart suffers. When ATP levels are normal, energy is supported, cellular activity increases, and the body thrives. One of the most important ways to sustain and build lifelong health is by producing and preserving ATP in the mitochondria.

Since learning about all of this more than 30 years ago through my study of nutrition and aging, I've been a committed "mitochon-driac," obsessed with the importance and care of these infinitesimal structures that churn out the energy that stokes each cell and thus, in sum, your heart and the rest of your body. I was taught very little about mitochondria in medical school, but I realized after years of clinical practice, that health and vitality relate directly to the health and vitality of the mitochondria. As they go, so go you. Their status is your status. Mitochondrial DNA—unlike nuclear DNA—has no defense mechanisms, so you must nurture and support these tiny structures.

To boost ATP, it's important to "fertilize" your mitochondria in order to counteract all the toxicity to which you are exposed in soci-ety. This concept works the same way as caring for a garden. You use natural fertilizers and then watch your plants grow and reach for the sun. As I've told my patients many times, you want to give similar loving care to your mitochondria so they stay healthy, vibrant, and long-lived.

One way to fertilize the mitochondria is with a nutrient called coenzyme Q10 (CoQ10). This vitamin-like substance plays a vital role in the production of energy at the cellular level. ATP can't be produced without CoQ10, which the body takes in from the foods we eat. Wild migratory salmon and sardines, as well as organ meats such as liver and heart contain the highest quantities of CoQ10. You can obtain this nutrient from supplements, too. The body cells also make CoQ10, which is referred to as "endogenous" (*endo* = inside) formation. The liver and kidneys assist the most in this production. CoQ10 is an incredibly important ingredient in your body's makeup.

I became aware of CoQ10 through an article that discussed how administering this nutrient is associated with stronger heart function. I immediately started to prescribe CoQ10 to any patient about to undergo open heart surgery. It wasn't long before I discovered that CoQ10 offered much, much more, and is, in fact, a true lifesaver.

One of my earliest clinical encounters with the power of this nutrient was with a patient named Joan, who was 34 when she came to see me. After giving birth to her second child, she suffered "postpartum cardiomyopathy." This is a very rare, life-threatening form of heart failure that can occur in a pregnant woman when the fetal circulatory system steals too many nutrients from her body. Consequently, while the baby gets the nutrition, the mother becomes malnourished. After the baby is delivered, the mother is at risk of suffering heart failure.

Joan went from doctor to doctor, hearing only that she needed a heart transplant or she would die. She was even placed on a heart transplant list.

Joan consulted with me, and I put her on CoQ10 for a few weeks. Her symptoms began to subside. I doubled the dosage twice, and she vastly improved. A year after being placed on the transplant list, she was informed that the medical facility had found a heart match for her.

Joan contacted me to report: "I feel fine. Should I get a heart transplant?"

"Follow your own intuition. I can't make that decision for you," I advised.

Joan refused the heart transplant and stayed on my plan. Today, she is almost 72 years old and still going strong.

Joan is just one of many cases I've had like this, in which fertilizing the mitochondria repairs and rejuvenates the heart. Over the years, I've helped avert heart transplants in dozens of patients by boosting their bodies—and theoretically, their mitochondria—with natural substances such as CoQ10.

I've had doctors call me to say how amazed they are that their patients are still alive and doing so well. To be sure, it wasn't just the food and supplements I recommended, but an overall plan of physical activity, stress reduction, and thinking positively that helped turn around declining hearts. But behind all that is the core issue: the quantity of ATP supported by targeted nutrients generated by your mitochondria to run your body—a program I call Metabolic Cardiology.

As the Teacher explained to Tommy, all sorts of toxins, from chemical and electric pollution to pharmaceutical drugs, assault the mitochondria and create dysfunction. This leads to DNA damage, tissue deterioration, and organ impairment—and that means impairment of any organ because every cell is connected to every other cell. Thousands of studies have now been published on mitochondria and the abnormal mitochondrial dynamics involved in diseases like Alzheimer's and Parkinson's, diabetes, obesity, autoimmune conditions, cancer, heart disease, migraine headaches, chronic fatigue syndrome, and even aging itself. More than 50 million people in the United States are said to be affected by conditions involving mitochondrial dysfunction.

As a young cardiologist, I was surprised to learn that widely used, everyday substances in the environment are toxic to the heart and can deplete the Vital Force. The very first case I encountered involved a young man (he was my own age at the time, 32!) who developed a wild, life-threatening arrhythmia while painting a windowless room in his house. It turned out that the paint was the toxin threatening his life! It was touch-and-go for more than a day before we finally pulled him out of the lethal arrhythmia and into a normal heart rhythm.

I'll never forget that case. It opened my awareness to a source of trouble that cardiologists-to-be were not taught about in medical school: There are toxins we encounter every single day that disrupt our bodies' functioning. The potential is real and often something right under your nose.

In fact, according to the American Academy of Environmental Medicine, there are some 90,000 chemicals commonly circulating in our lives, with perhaps 10 to 15 percent of us believed to be reactive to one thing or another, even natural substances.

Over the years, it became obvious to me that anybody can be reactive to almost anything in the environment—food, pesticides, solvents, mold, airborne particulates, air fresheners, and, of course, the medications doctors use to treat symptoms—and that reactions are extremely individual. One person may have an allergic reaction; another might develop fatigue or a headache, and another an arrhythmia.

Acute exposures aside, doctors specializing in environmental illness often talk about the "total load" of environmental stressors, or insults, that result in symptoms. Think of your immune system as a barrel with a specific capacity. That capacity can shrink or enlarge depending on your toxic exposure at a given time, whether to physical toxins or to toxic psychological stress. You may or may not be aware of the specific toxins filling up your barrel and only know that something is wrong when the barrel spills over and you develop symptoms.

Some time ago, I developed a list of what I consider the most toxic substances in our daily life. I share them with you here, along with the same advice I gave to my patients. You obviously can't dodge all of these bullets. We live in a sea of chemicals. But do try to avoid or minimize exposure to as many of them as you can in order to keep your barrel from spilling over. Here is a list of the 10 common toxins we encounter in everyday living and, in my opinion, how to avoid them.

1. **Pesticides.** Many of our fruits and vegetables are sprayed with pesticides, and we end up ingesting the residues. To avoid pesticides and other additives in food, eat washed organic produce. Researchers have found that organic fruits and vegetables are much, much lower in pesticide residue, and perhaps higher in natural antioxidants, compared with nonorganic produce.

   Avoid using toxic pesticide products in your home and yard, too, and seek out other, more natural solutions for pest control. An example: A mixture of ¼ cup lemon juice, 1 tablespoon vanilla extract, and 15 drops of lavender oil, and enough water to fill a 16-ounce spray bottle makes a superior mosquito repellant.

2. **Prescription drugs.** Citing the Institute of Medicine, the US Food and Drug Administration (FDA) states that each year, more than two million adverse drug reactions (ADRs) occur, and these reactions account for 100,000 annual deaths, making ADRs the "fourth leading cause of death." ADRs are largely preventable, and side effects often compound the original problem drugs are taken for. Unfortunately, side effects are often dismissed by doctors and grossly underreported. Many pharmaceutical drugs are mitochrondrial-toxic and can deplete the body of nutrients, which is something that doctors never tell you. Many drugs are too strong.

   Often, natural alternatives can help get at the underlying causes of chronic problems and minimize or eliminate risky medication usage. These alternatives include eating organic, nutritious food; taking nutritional supplements; engaging in regular exercise; and following a good stress-reduction method. However, if you want to stop taking a drug or ease back on it, always consult your doctor first.

3. **Alcohol.** Moderate intake—one drink daily for a woman, two for men—may have therapeutic value, but imbibing more than that is asking for trouble. Liver destruction and nutritional deficiencies are among the many possible consequences of heavy drinking. Excess alcohol causes nutritional deficiencies. Alcohol breaks down into aldehyde, a substance that damages cellular membranes and causes premature aging.

4. **Indoor and outdoor pollution.** Air pollution is no joke; it does damage to cells and organs over time. Use an air purifier, at least in the rooms where you spend the most time, to reduce dust and other particulate matter. Install a water-filter system to purify the

beverage your body needs the most: water. Be aware of sensitivities to outdoor chemicals, pollen, and mold. Don't walk, jog, or bike in the city during rush hour.

5. **Cigarette smoke.** Smoking is a cardinal sin against health. Lung cancer aside, this habit is the most destructive for the heart and nearly every other organ in the body. Each puff carries a toxic payload of chemicals and carcinogens, including nicotine (used as a natural pesticide for hundreds of years), carbon monoxide, ammonia, arsenic, cadmium, lead, and formaldehyde, to name just a few of the 600 ingredients. If you smoke and recognize that you need to stop, seek help through your physician or a credible smoking-cessation program.

6. **Formaldehyde.** This chemical is also used in the production of fertilizer, paper, plywood, particleboard, and urea-formaldehyde resins; as a preservative in some foods; and in many products used around the house, such as paints, antiseptics, medicines, cosmetics, furniture, carpets, and cabinetry. Formaldehyde can irritate the skin, throat, nose, and eyes; high-level exposure, most commonly related to the resins industry, is linked to some cancers. In 2006, the International Agency for Research on Cancer, a branch of the World Health Organization, classified formaldehyde as a "known human carcinogen," and the US government followed suit in 2011. The primary way you can be exposed to formaldehyde is by breathing air containing it. Open windows to bring fresh air indoors. Also, reduce your dependency on dry cleaning, since the process used to keep clothes wrinkle-free often involves the use of a formaldehyde resin. Air out any clothes or other products that may have been exposed to formaldehyde.

7. **Personal-hygiene products.** We smear and spray our skin with all sorts of creams, sunscreens, lotions, soaps, perfumes, and what-not.

The best strategies are to opt for natural products whenever possible and use personal care products minimally, because what goes on the skin also can go into the skin . . . and into the body. That means multiple chemicals. Most deodorants, for instance, contain aluminum to prevent perspiration; aluminum is known to cause DNA alterations, and daily dermal exposure may, over time, lead to breast cancer. Another example is antibacterial soap, in either bar or liquid form. Americans scoop up nearly $1 billion worth of these products a year, even though studies show that they are no more effective than regular soap and water at reducing the spread of germs. These products contain two active ingredients—triclocarban and triclosan—that have been found in experiments to disrupt reproductive hormone activity and interfere with cell signaling activities, including in the brain and heart. Buyer beware!

For those personal-care products you can't live without, the Environmental Working Group (EWG—www.ewg.org) has established Skin Deep, an electronic product database through which you can learn about the known chemical toxicity of almost 64,000 cosmetic products. Although labels don't give you all the information you need to decide whether products are safe, reading them carefully is a good place to start. Choose products with the fewest ingredients and chemicals, and avoid chemical fragrances altogether.

Good alternatives to perfumes and fragrances are essential oils. For sunscreen, apply zinc oxide. It is the best, safest, and most nonabsorbable sunblock you can use.

8. **Petrochemicals.** Surprise! Derivatives of petrochemicals are found in most processed food, personal-care, and cleaning products. Households are literally brimming with the stuff that has the potential to increase your risks of short- and long-term health issues, including cancer. Try to minimize exposure. For sure, cut

down on processed food as much as possible, and eat organic. Be aware that solvents can cause lung and throat irritation, and furniture polish may be flammable and can cause serious injury if accidentally swallowed. (Avoid products, when possible, with the word *danger* on the label.) The EWG is also an excellent resource for learning more about petrochemicals and other toxins in your everyday life.

9. **Heavy metals.** Lead from dust, dirt, old house paint, batteries, new toys, and even water flowing through lead-lined pipes can increase the risks of a number of health issues. The nervous systems of young children and the unborn are most vulnerable. Cadmium is another toxic metal, and exposure can contribute to hypertension, among other things. Cigarette smoke is a common source, but cadmium is also found in batteries, pigments, metal coatings, plastics, and fertilizers. Mercury, one of the most potent mitochondrial toxins, is pervasive in freshwater fish and in large seawater fish, such as shark, tuna, swordfish, orange roughy, large halibut, and grouper.

10. **Phthalates and bisphenol A (BPA).** Both of these common compounds, used in plastics, are under ongoing scrutiny because of potential health risks to humans, including reproductive risks. Phthalates are used in soft plastics, and BPA in hard plastics and food can linings. Both are commonly found in products ranging from cosmetics, soaps, and lotions to food packaging and water bottles. If you're a dialysis patient, hemophiliac, or blood transfusion recipient, you're at the highest risk of exposure to phthalates through the tubing or containers made with this compound. The FDA recommends certain steps to minimize exposure of patients to medical devices that contain phthalates, including use of alternative devices for certain procedures. Other people at high risk are painters, printers, and workers exposed to phthalates during the manufacture, formulation, and processing of plastics.

Although there are many concerns over potential risks of BPA, the FDA has not banned it and has deemed it safe at low doses. I have seen research describing an association between higher levels of BPA and risks of high blood pressure and coronary artery disease; however, the degree of the chemical's influence on health is far from clear. My advice is to simply reduce your exposure and steer clear of plastic containers whenever you can. Avoid canned foods as much as possible, and drink water out of glass bottles or containers.

In addition to all these actions, another way to protect yourself against toxins and fortify your Vital Force is through targeted nutritional supplementation. This fertilizes your mitochondria, thus strengthening your Vital Force. Along with CoQ10, there are three other ATP-boosting nutrients: magnesium, carnitine, and d-ribose. Magnesium is essential for metabolism of food and release of energy; it is also important in preserving the DNA in the mitochondria. Carnitine transports fatty acids to the mitochondria and helps remove toxins. Finally, d-ribose is a naturally occurring sugar derivative of ATP and can help keep mitochondria functioning at a higher level. I call these four nutrients the "Awesome Foursome"; they are the foundation of my Metabolic Cardiology plan.

To that plan, however, I add a fifth element: omega-3 fatty acid supplements. Omega-3's compounds are additional favorites of mine because of the many benefits for the heart and overall health. Here are just a few perks of supplementing with omega-3s. They:

▓ Increase HDL (the good cholesterol)

▓ Decrease triglycerides and normalize blood pressure

▓ Help neutralize harmful effects of Lp(a)—a protein in the blood that is a risk factor for heart disease

- Reduce arterial wall inflammation and improve endothelial function (Endothelial cells line our arteries and are the major producer of nitric oxide [NO], a molecule responsible for relaxing the blood vessels and maintaining healthy blood flow.)

- Make blood less sticky and less likely to form clots

- Prevent plaque ruptures

- Prevent and ease cardiac arrhythmias

Omega-3 supplements come in plant- or marine-based forms. Plant-based products are made from flaxseed and chia. My preference over the years has been marine-derived products because they directly supply the beneficial omega-3 fats, eicosapentaenoic acid (EPA) and docosahexaenoic acid (DHA). Flaxseeds and chia contain the fatty acid alpha-linolenic acid, which has to be converted to EPA and DHA in the body—a process that requires a lot of energy. Thus, it makes sense to obtain EPA and DHA directly so that you conserve the body's energy.

For years, I recommended fish oil, but more recently I switched to squid oil because harvesting squid has less impact on the marine ecology. Squid oil also has a higher concentration of DHA, which has added benefits for eye, heart, and brain tissue. Moreover, DHA has a greater ability to lower blood pressure than EPA and may improve learning and memory function among individuals over 55 with age-related declines in brain function.

I take all five as supplements every day, and I also eat foods that are high in these nutrients. The best foods for CoQ10 are wild migratory salmon and sardines; for carnitine, the best source is lamb. For magnesium, consume nuts, seeds (especially pumpkin seeds), leafy greens, beans, and figs. You can't get ribose from food, so a supplement is your best line of offense. You find omega-3s in wild migratory salmon, tuna, and flaxseeds.

The daily dosages I suggest are:

50–100 milligrams of CoQ10 (preferably in softgels)

200–400 milligrams of magnesium

200–400 milligrams of l-carnitine

1 teaspoon of d-ribose

1–2 grams of omega-3 supplements, taken in divided doses

If you are physically compromised, especially with cardiac issues, you will need higher doses of these supplements; discuss this with your physician. For more clarity or in-depth discussion about my Metabolic Cardiology program, I suggest you read the latest edition of *The Sinatra Solution: Metabolic Cardiology,* Basic Health Publications, 2011.

I can't tell you how many of my patients have reported that, by taking the mitochondria-supporting measures prescribed to heal the body, they saw other illnesses improve as well, including macular degeneration (the most common form of blindness in the world; runs in my own family), migraine, diabetes, digestive stress, and musculoskeletal disorders. In my mind, fertilizing your mitochondria is the best way to prevent aging (power blackouts) as you get older.

I also recommend deep and rhythmic breathing to fight the toxins that deplete our Vital Force. You see, the respiratory system helps detoxify the body. In addition to disposing of carbon dioxide, our respiratory system includes several protective mechanisms to prevent infiltration of toxins from the air we breathe. Our first line of defense is the nose, which contains hairs that filter foreign substances. Our bronchial tubes are lined with more hairs, called cilia, which facilitate the upward movement of mucus to enable coughing, sneezing, and swallowing.

Although unpleasant, mucus helps us expel unwanted substances by acting as a fly strip of sorts. When we have colds and take over-the-counter medications to suppress mucus production, we may actually prolong sickness by disabling our bodies' natural abilities to fight back.

Lymphatic tissues lining the walls of the throat, trachea, and bronchioles also help rid the lungs of health-threatening invaders. Lymph nodes are clusters of cells that contain immune cells to fight the foreign substances they collect. The adenoids, located at the top of the throat, are lymph tissues, and the tonsils are localized lymphatic tissues within the throat. (Sometimes doctors remove adenoids or tonsils that have become infected and enlarged enough to hinder the respiration process.)

Employing various detoxification pathways when sick can help us avoid lymphatic overload. For example, sweating in a sauna is an excellent way to eliminate heavy metals, toxins, petrochemicals, insecticides, and pesticides that reside in our subcutaneous fat. Several of my patients strongly believe that they "cured" themselves by sweating out such toxins in infrared and Swedish saunas. In addition, taking a day or two of rest and allowing a sickness to run its course may be just what the doctor ordered.

Finally, it is important to know whether your Vital Force is strong or waning. One of the most accurate ways to measure your Vital Force is through this simple method: taking your body temperature. It requires an enormous amount of ATP to generate a normal body temperature of 98.6°F. If body temperature drops below normal, that means cellular energy has begun to drop, setting the stage for a bodily takeover by viruses, bacteria, fungi, and other dangerous diseases.

On the other hand, never be afraid of having a slight fever. A fever is one of the body's protective mechanisms and can effectively destroy certain microbes, while protecting against infection and stimulating the immune system. The hotter your body temperature, the less likely it is that germs, other invaders, and even cancer cells will survive.

What Tommy's Teacher told him about the self-healing wisdom

of the body is absolutely true. The human body completely regenerates itself over time. The cells in your gastrointestinal tract are replaced once a year; your red blood cells, every 120 days. And 40 percent of your heart cells are replaced over a lifetime. As long as you treat it well, your body can stay in a constant state of renewal and resurrection and has an innate wisdom to heal itself. Treating it well means giving it the resources it needs (nutrition, the Awesome Foursome, water, positive thoughts, and love) and avoiding what is toxic (sugar, pollutants, and negativity).

By taking these actions, you buy time for the body's intrinsic stem cells—special cells that replace diseased or damaged cells with healthy ones—to take over and drive the regeneration of the body. That, in a nutshell, is how self-healing takes place and how your Vital Force maintains the life—and the aliveness—in your body.

Applying the Revelation of
VITAL FORCE

We looked at actions you can take to protect and foster your Vital Force. Consider personalizing those actions in a plan that makes sense to you. For example:

- I will focus on renewing my Vital Force by caring for my body in a way that allows healing. I will make better nutritional choices daily, taking targeted supplements to support my cells' ability to rejuvenate and regenerate. I will nurture and "fertilize" mitochondria with foods and supplements containing CoQ10, magnesium, L-carnitine, and d-ribose to support my Vital Force energy for cellular renewal. I will also take omega-3 fats.

- I will recognize and respect the self-healing powers of my body. It contains its own innate healing wisdom and vast defenses that can overcome illness, prolong life, and work health miracles. I will let go of anything that does not support those powers.

- I will become more aware of potential toxins in my environment. I will buy pesticide-free foods and products that are safe for my home. I will avoid cigarette smoke and be more aware of sensitivities to outdoor chemicals, pollen, and mold. I will use an air purifier, at least in rooms where I spend the most time, to reduce dust and other particulate matter. Caring for my body, my home, and my immediate environment in this way allows for healing and a vibrant Vital Force.

- I will support my Vital Force with rhythmic deep breathing. Part of that support will include performing this exercise at least five minutes every day.

Applying the Revelation of Vital Force (continued)

- Sit erect (but not stiff) in a straight chair with a pillow placed between your shoulder blades. Remove your shoes. Place your feet firmly on the floor or, weather permitting, barefoot on the Earth outside.

- Gently open your mouth. Let your jaw hang softly.

- Breathe in and out through your nose, with your awareness on each inhalation and exhalation.

- Place your hands over your navel and, with your eyes closed, feel your abdomen rise under your hands.

When our breathing is calm and slowed down, our Vital Force is nurtured.

CHAPTER
6

THE REVELATION
of GROUNDING

AS MY TEACHER SHARES all of this with me, I feel like a kid, with endless curiosity. I'm beginning to see that we all have within us the power to change the conditions and energies in our lives through connection, faith, and our Vital Force. But I want to know more about health and healing; now that I am beginning to understand how influenced the mind, body, and spirit are by each other, I want to know more about how I can help them work in harmony. My eagerness tells me that I seem to be a much better student in Heaven than I was as a schoolkid on Earth.

As if sensing my curiosity, my Teacher begins to reveal more about these things. He says something that instantly gets my attention.

I give my people ways to heal, but they do not use them.

What can he mean?
My Teacher then describes the Revelation of Grounding.

The Earth has a vibration that heals your body. You can connect to this healing force by grounding to the Earth. This means walking barefoot each day for one-half hour, touching and embracing living trees, which are rooted in the Earth. You can also ground by swimming in the sea for a few minutes each day. You can meditate or pray as you ground yourself to the grass or the sea or the sand. The more you ground to the planet, the more you will heal yourself from everyday radiation, toxicity, inflammation, stress, sleeping problems, and pain.

You mean I can just go outside, kick off my shoes, and plug into Earth's vibration for healing?

Yes, and you will also protect yourself from electronic bombardment from your technologies. These unseen forces affect the body's own electromagnetic field and lower vibration. This toxicity allows negative energy to enter into organs of the body. The organs become susceptible to invasion.

By raising the body's vibration through grounding, you will increase the efficiency of the body's immune system, circulatory system, and overall health.

As my Teacher reveals this information, we're on the top of a hill. I look below and see a beautiful crystal-clear lake, encircled by rolling hills with deep green grass and abundant flowers. The lake is calm and serene. Like everything else there, the water emanates a conscious light and love. What a beautiful place to learn about the Earth's healing power.

My Teacher sees and senses my awe.

Water is the life of the planet. All human beings have a significant amount of water within them, so water is life itself. The water on Earth has its own frequency and vibration. It nourishes, cleanses, and protects all the inhabitants of the planet. Without water, your species and all others would perish and disappear from Earth's varied ecosystems. The flowers, the trees and vegetation, and water in all of its forms contribute to raising the vibration of the planet.

Seeing this heavenly environment and listening to these teachings makes me think how wonderful Earth would be if our rivers and streams and oceans were that clean, clear, and soothing! I feel so sad that we have treated our home, our planet, so poorly. I wonder what will happen if we go on polluting Earth.

You are right. Unfortunately, the planet is becoming more toxic. Plastics tossed carelessly into the environment are a huge problem, as are prescription medications. You may not realize it, but they find their way into the oceans and are ingested by fish, which are then consumed by people throughout the world. There must be more respect for the other creatures and beings you share your planet with and for the beautiful planet Earth.

Yet, my Teacher assures me that despite the abuse to the environment, our physical Earth is still strong and will stay that way as long as people continue to respect it.

Mother Earth has a very special place in God's universe because of her ability to rid people of accumulated negative energy. This will be true as long as the Earth does not become polluted beyond repair. If the Earth's toxicity reaches a certain level, then, like a toxic body, the planet's systems will cease to be able to function as they are meant to. Her ability to support and nourish life will be severely diminished. The Earth will no longer be a safe haven. Those who do not consider the needs of the planet they reside upon, who use her precious resources selfishly and thoughtlessly, giving no thought to replenishment, and those

who do not nurture her will find themselves homeless. What
humanity continues to do will not be undone.

To be sure, we have become careless about our beautiful home,
Earth. I think about myself; I recycle; I don't litter. But that's hardly
enough. There must be more I can do to help our planet!

My Teacher responds to my thoughts.

Yes, my son, each of you has a great responsibility to care
for what you have been given: your life; your mind, body, and
spirit; your family and friends; your gifts and special talents—
and your planet.

I think hard about this. I had never thought of the Earth as a
living design of God or considered the fact that we coexist with her
in a symbiotic relationship. But now that my Teacher has said it, it
seems so clear. Earth supports every species of life and has been
sustaining us since the beginning of time. The health of the planet
is connected to the health of humanity.

Yet we've been destroying her and, in doing so, destroying our
own survival as a people! We need to take responsibility for Earth's
health, too, and bring about a new experience of living on this planet
without pollution, soil- and crop-destroying farming methods, or
anything that has been holding us—and the Earth—back from really
fulfilling our health and healing potential.

After hearing the Revelation of Grounding, I desire even more to
take care of the Earth, respect her, and do my part to not pollute or
use products that hurt her. I feel grateful to Mother Earth for the
gift of health she provides if we just connect with her and honor
her. She reflects the beauty in the world and reminds me that by
taking care of her, we take care of ourselves. I want to be outdoors
more; immerse myself in nature; enjoy the oceans, lakes, and rivers; and make space in my life to bask in and tap into the Earth's
healing power.

The Sinatra Prescription on Grounding

I was both astounded and touched to learn of this revelation from Tommy. I have long been convinced that the body is healthier when we have more physical contact with the natural energetic field of the Earth. I have been intensely involved in grounding research for years and written extensively about it. Grounding (also referred to as Earthing) means connecting your body directly to this field and experiencing the benefits of connection with the electric fields of the Earth.

This is easy to do. My recommendation is to ground at least 150 minutes a week. You can do that by going barefoot while gardening, camping, hiking, or walking on the beach or by swimming in the ocean—there are so many ways to connect to the natural world. When outdoors, wearing thin-soled, plain leather shoes will let you make contact with the Earth's natural vibration. Rubber soles like those of tennis sneakers or the neoprene found in running shoes will keep you disconnected from the Earth. You can even sleep, work, or relax indoors on special conductive sheets or mats connected to the Earth with wires plugged into a grounded wall outlet or a ground rod outside.

Although studied scientifically in the last decade, grounding dates back to prehistoric ages. Since the dawn of time, humans have walked barefoot and slept on the ground, oblivious to the subtle energetic signals underfoot that research now shows help regulate the body's intricate mechanisms. Healers in many cultures throughout history knew of the natural healing endowment of the Earth, though not in electrical terms.

In the Bahamas, I once learned from a bush medicine woman how to use the ocean's tides to accelerate healing. This knowledge was a form of grounding. She told me: "On an outgoing tide, dig your heels into the sand up to your ankles. Swing your arms back and forth to facilitate lymph flow. Then bend at your knees as you swing your arms all the way forward and all the way back as you feel the surge of the tide."

This made perfect sense to me, because our electrical body is 70 percent water. The surging outgoing tide can literally pull toxic energies from the body.

If you're too weak to try this exercise, sit in a chair at the water's edge and place your lower legs in the water. The combination of the magnetic energy of the earth, the minerals in the sand and sea, and the tide surge creates a healing vibration that diffuses throughout the entire body. This exercise is a perfect solution for quelling inflammation.

Humans, as well as all living beings and plants, are bioelectric life-forms in constant interaction with the environment. Collectively, cells form a living matrix through which the body conducts electrical impulses. Our cells resonate to particular frequencies and are in continual transmission and receipt of energy. For instance, we owe the heart's rhythmic beating in part to electrical impulses. Our nervous and immune systems, as well as muscular activity, also involve electrical currents. Electric fields regulate the movement of nutrients and water into our cells.

Biochemists frequently refer to the sodium/calcium pumps providing energy transfer into the heart cells. We look like flesh and bone but we really are electrical beings. The natural energy of the Earth supports the entire electrical cellular framework of the body.

With modern life, heavily insulated homes and buildings and rubber- and plastic-soled shoes have largely disconnected us from the Earth's healing energy—a disconnect that may be an overlooked cause in the steep rise of diseases, fatigue, stress, and poor sleep that plague contemporary societies.

One of my greatest discoveries in more than 40 years of clinical practice is the positive, healing impact that grounding has on blood viscosity, or thickness. When blood thickens like ketchup, it can promote blood clotting and inflammation. Our group of investigators showed that connecting to Mother Earth's energy—also known as the Schumann resonance and measured at 7.83 hertz—caused red cells to repel one another with greater force, thus making the blood's consistency more like red wine; this meant that more oxygen was being delivered to the tissues. In essence, by increasing the velocity of blood and improving oxygen delivery, grounding assuages the fires of inflammation. It puts the body into a healthy state.

Since highly thick blood, with inflamed blood vessels, is the cardinal cardiovascular risk factor for heart disease, it makes sense to ground. In my opinion, Earthing/grounding will reduce cardiovascular risk by connecting our bioelectric nature to that of the Earth.

Electrons move through the body via healing channels called meridians, which are stimulated largely by pressure at various points on the body. There is one very powerful point that just happens to be in the middle of the bottom of the foot—a point known to acupuncturists as Kidney 1 (KI 1). When you walk barefoot, you first press down on the KI 1 point. This activates the entire meridian that runs up your leg, over your back, through your kidneys, and up to your neck, terminating in the roof of your mouth, and you increase the flow of healing electrons to virtually every part of your body. It's a well-known fact that the surface of the Earth possesses a limitless supply of electrons, constantly replenished by lightning strikes and solar radiation. When allowed to flow into our bodies, these electrons work like antioxidants, disarming the free radicals that make us sick or age us.

Just think: God designed the foot so ingeniously that you and I can contact the Earth at the precise anatomical point that triggers healing!

As Tommy journeyed through Heaven, his Teacher told him about chakras. In contrast to meridians, these are a different interpretation of how energy flows through the body. Chakras are energy centers located throughout the body that comprise seven major points along the body's midline corresponding to specific organs, glands, and functions. Chakras constantly rotate and pulsate, drawing energy into the body. If any one of the chakras is blocked, the energy cannot flow, causing emotional and physical problems. One way to prevent blockages is to ground on a regular basis and let the Earth's energy open up the chakras and promote the flow of healing energy throughout the body.

Tommy's Teacher emphasized something else to him that modern-day scientists have only recently discovered: Grounding is an excellent way to protect the body from the wireless radiation and electromagnetic fields generated by electrical and wireless devices. Some people cannot tolerate these now ubiquitous emissions. Their hearts and brains, which have electrical systems of their own, may be affected.

A study reported in the journal *Atmospheric Environment* in August 2007 described how electromagnetic waves (EMW) emitted from computers, cell phones, Wi-Fi, and common household devices can trigger asthma, flu, and other respiratory problems. How, exactly? The research team of British scientists noted that electrical fields can charge invisible, ultrafine particles in the air, such as viruses, allergens, bacteria, and other toxins, keeping them airborne indefinitely. As a result, they are easily—and constantly—inhaled.

Further, in 2015, the World Health Organization's International Agency for Research on Cancer issued an alert that electromagnetic radiation from mobile phones and other wireless devices constitutes a probable human carcinogen.

Many people with hard-to-diagnose illnesses could benefit from understanding how cellular and cordless phones, cell phone towers, and Wi-Fi can and do cause breakdowns in numerous areas of the body. The invisible waves emitted are potentially harmful and impossible to completely eliminate, so countering that exposure with the Earth's natural vibrations is important. One of my special concerns is the relentless barrage of wireless technology that has exploded into daily living and its potentially hazardous effects on our health.

My family and I try to rely as little as possible on cellular and wireless technology. I feel "different" when I am exposed to these things. This has fostered an awareness that some people can be "electrically sensitive."

In 2012, assisted by other researchers, I published a review study on the health implications of grounding in the *Journal of Environmental and Public Health*. We reviewed and summarized more than 15 studies on grounding, as well as many others on the effect of the Earth's electrons on health. Basically, what we concluded from our review is that grounding helps improve cardiovascular, respiratory, digestive, nervous, and immune system function by restoring the body's natural internal electrical stability and rhythms. It also restores the body's healing potential. This study, along with my more than 10 years of research and observations, revealed that daily grounding activity can, for many:

- Decrease inflammation as well as assuage its physical symptoms

- Reduce or eliminate chronic pain

- Improve sleep

- Increase energy

- Thin blood and improve blood pressure and blood flow

- Relieve muscle tension and headaches

- Lessen hormonal and menstrual symptoms

- Speed healing, even after surgery, and prevent bedsores

- Alleviate or eliminate jet lag

▩ Protect the body against potentially health-disturbing environmental electromagnetic fields (EMFs)

▩ Accelerate recovery from intense athletic activity

▩ Balance the autonomic nervous system by decreasing sympathetic and increasing parasympathetic nervous activity: When dealing with challenges and stressful situations, we use our sympathetic nervous system and expend energy. When we're calm and relaxed, our parasympathetic nervous system kicks in, so the body can repair and restore itself.

Grounding may also boost your mood. In a first-of-its-kind study, researchers at the University of California, Irvine, tested 40 adults to see if grounding could improve mood. Part of the group grounded for one hour; the others did not ground. The participants' moods were assessed on a special scale before and after the experiment. Those who grounded reported pleasant and positive moods, while the others had no improvement. The researchers reported their findings in the April 2015 issue of *Psychological Reports*.

Everybody benefits from grounding but in different ways. The positive results can come quickly and dramatically, such as less pain and better sleep, or subtly and gradually over time. Often, people who are very ill or saddled with various symptoms notice a dramatic difference. Someone who has radiant health and sleeps well may not feel the differences so dramatically, but connecting to the Earth helps preserve and perpetuate that good health. I sincerely regard grounding as a simple, natural form of antiaging and preventive medicine, whether the benefits are obvious or subtle.

Through the simple and powerful method of grounding, we can remember our connection to nature and, in doing so, reclaim aspects of our health that need rejuvenation. Where there is Earth, there is healing.

Applying the Revelation of
GROUNDING

Grounding is one of the easiest and most uplifting ways to improve your health and overcome issues that may be related to electromagnetic sensitivities in the environment. Here are some action steps to help you personalize the recommendations discussed above.

* I will place my feet on the grass, soil, sand, concrete, or brick at least a half hour daily and walk barefoot on the Earth. I will seek out other ways to ground and immerse myself in nature: swimming in the ocean, a lake, or a river; hiking in the mountains; or lying under the stars.

* I will reduce the time I spend toggled to devices and electronic ways of communicating. Instead of searching for things on the Internet, I will look for ways to be with nature. I will write down a list of changes I'm willing to make and cross them off as I reduce my exposure. Some examples:

  * Limit the number and duration of my cell phone calls, and use a speakerphone whenever possible.

  * Throw away my cordless phones and use plug-in versions, such as landlines.

  * Turn off my cell phone when not in use and stow it away from my body.

  * Unplug electrical equipment when not in use.

  * Turn off my router at night or use a wired-only router.

  * Use grounding or Earthing pads under my laptop to shield my body from electrical charges.

Applying the Revelation of Grounding (continued)

- Move my clock or radio away from my bed so EMFs aren't directed at my head.

- Stand back at least 30 feet from my microwave when it is cooking. Or reduce my dependence on microwave cooking.

- Avoid living near cellular towers and high-tension power lines, if possible and feasible.

- I will use my grounding time to cultivate an appreciative relationship with Mother Earth. When I can listen to nature through the simplest of acts—walking among trees and plants, connecting with the mineral-rich sand at the seashore, or watching birds—I will notice the rhythm of life and feel a sense of belonging to the natural world. I will actively express gratitude for the healing gifts Mother Earth provides.

CHAPTER
7

THE REVELATION
of THE BODY TEMPLE

DURING MY TIME WITH my Teacher, I observe that no one is eating, not even the animals. I haven't been hungry here. My stomach isn't even grumbling for a meal.

This feels odd to me because I love food. I'm a meat-and-potatoes man. Pizza is my other favorite. And I eat sugar, a lot of it, especially when I want a fast snack. I never paid much attention to diets or nutrition.

My Teacher seems to know this. When he sees me reflecting curiously on the role of food in this place, he gives me a lesson in nutrition that is simply unlike anything I've ever heard. It is called the Revelation of the Body Temple. It will change me, how I look at food, and what I put in my body.

When you are in the physical body, the amount of food you eat and the kind of food you eat affect the body's vibrational

*rate. For example, too much sugar, too many chemicals or dyes,
or bacteria in food or drink lowers vibration. Alcohol and drugs
also negatively affect the body's vibration.*

*During the digestive process, your body cannot process tox-
ins. Eating too much food lowers your body's ability to detoxify,
which is why people who consume less food are generally
healthier and live longer.*

I've certainly been known to take second helpings—and then
some! I never drank alcohol, but I definitely love food, and not the
green, leafy kind!

I'm curious about the dangers of refined sugars, the kind you find
in table sugar, soft drinks, and other sweet foods. I want to know if
the unhealthy effects of sugar I've read about are true.

*Let's just say refined sugar is the enemy of a healthy body.
It robs the body of nutrition and lowers the white blood count
for hours. This allows the immune system to become overrun
with toxins such as metals, fungi, parasites, bacteria, and
viruses.*

*Refined sugar will initially provide a quick burst of energy,
but soon that energy dissipates. You are left feeling tired, even
lethargic, and depressed. Consuming sugar causes chronic
inflammation in your entire body and leads to issues with the
heart, liver, and kidneys.*

I think about what happens when I eat lots of sugar or carbs. It's
delicious in the moment, but I usually feel bad the next day. Sugar,
especially—it makes me feel good when I eat it, but I've noticed that I
get depressed the day after a sugar binge. My sweet tooth certainly
hasn't helped my weight, either. Sometimes I'll grab a candy bar for the
energy boost while working a late job. My Teacher continues the lesson.

*In simple terms, the physical body exists to house the spirit.
Think of the body as a house or temple around the soul. It is*

your job to keep the house clean, healthy, and loving, so your spirit can grow and thrive. The spirit or soul is an indestructible energy that lives with or without a physical body, but the body cannot live without its spirit.

Whoever said that "you are what you eat" wasn't kidding!

I realize that everything my Teacher has shown and told me until this point is about what makes humans sick and what makes us well on Earth. It's astonishing to me how many resources and gifts are in our power; we spend countless hours and dollars looking for miracle cures, following crazy programs, and bemoaning how hard it is to find health and happiness. But what my Teacher is telling me is that the real miracles are all well within our reach, right there in the natural world, if only we would open our eyes and see.

My Teacher's explanations make me understand in a new way that the body is a gift from God. He created these temples—our bodies—and gave them to us to take care of to the best of our ability.

How easy it is to forget this! So often, we take our bodies for granted and abuse them with bad food, alcohol, drugs, smoking, lack of exercise, and other unhealthy choices. It's sad. I know people who smoke, then wonder why they get cancer, or eat the wrong foods and wonder why their arteries become blocked, or become alcoholics and wonder why their livers are failing. Sickness is self-created!

The choices we make, including what we eat, clearly influence the quality of our lives. We can make ourselves weak and eventually sick, or we can lead our lives in a way that makes us healthy and strong. God has already given us everything we need, but it's up to us to actually use all of His blessings!

When I think of how I've spent my time on Earth, I realize that caring for my body hasn't been much of a priority. I've let work responsibilities, family obligations, and stress get in the way of taking care of me. I long for a chance to reset my priorities and live my life by these new, healthier, more self-loving principles!

There's a lot I can do in my own life to be healthy, and this reve-lation reminds me how precious my body is. I don't want to be pas-sive anymore about my health choices. I no longer want to abuse this gift from God—my body.

Hearing me figure things out in my head, my Teacher seems pleased that I'm connecting the dots.

> *Every choice, every decision you make in life, affects you positively or negatively. Remember that each of you is born with free will, which is a gift from God that allows you to choose your path and the pace of your own personal and spiritual evolution.*

As I listen to my Teacher, I can't help thinking about how much of a wake-up call I've needed when it comes to taking care of my body. But I'm here in Heaven and probably dead. Still, I wonder if maybe my Teacher intends for me to go back to Earth and have a second chance to take better care of myself.

The Sinatra Prescription on the Body Temple

It's true, as Tommy's Teacher described, that our choices have an enormous impact on our physical and mental health. It seems like it should be so easy for us to make good choices, but, of course, mil-lions and millions of us struggle to follow this important wisdom.

As Tommy discovered in Heaven, food is definitely medicine, so long as it is the proper type of food—natural and organic, preferably. I'll talk about those choices shortly, but first I want to address certain foods that are, by their very nature, toxic, which means that they can cause harm in any quantity but especially if consumed too frequently. My personal hit list of toxic foods includes the following five.

Trans fats. These are the harmful, man-made, partially hydro-genated fats that food processors use to prolong shelf life in an estimated 75 percent of the food eaten in the standard American diet. They appear everywhere, including margarine, most packaged baked goods, fried snacks, frozen products such as fish sticks and french fries, microwave popcorn, commercial salad dressings, and pancake mixes.

Trans fats are associated with increased oxidative damage to cell membranes, injury that kindles inflammation, disease, and age-related changes. They promote all sorts of heart problems and are believed to contribute to diabetes, cancer, autoimmune disease, tendon and bone degeneration, and problems with fertility and growth.

In 2006, the FDA began requiring food manufacturers to list trans fat content on labels, and in 2013 the agency proposed that partially hydrogenated oils are no longer "generally recognized as safe" for use in food (this proposal has yet to be made official). In response to increased public consciousness about trans fat content in food and its health implications, some manufacturers have changed their recipes—some for the better, and some for the "still unhealthy, but not any worse."

For example, many commercial brands of peanut butter once contained trans fats, which gave the products their characteristic silky-smooth texture; now most, if not all, brands have replaced partially hydrogenated oils with fully hydrogenated ones to avoid including trans fat content on the label. Fully hydrogenated fats—made chemically through a process called *interesterification*, which transforms unsaturated fats into saturated ones—can still contain some trans fat and are not "safe." If you like to eat peanut butter, opt for a "natural" variety, free of any hydrogenated oils or other suspect ingredients, such as corn syrup, sugar, and polyunsaturated oils.

Not only are trans fats found in foods with partially hydrogenated oils, as well as some fully hydrogenated oils, but they also occur as a result of frying: The high heat leads to the partial decomposition of fat and the formation of toxic by-products. Read labels and avoid processed products with any trans fat content whatsoever. Be aware, however, that even if a label says "zero" trans fat, a small amount is still allowed. This is one reason to minimize the amount of processed food in your life, despite the convenience. Don't cook with polyunsaturated vegetable oils. They break down too rapidly and form trans fats.

Cooked meats. Cooking meat at high temperature, such as pan frying or grilling over an open flame, can form chemicals that may increase your cancer risk. The chemicals are called heterocyclic amines and polycyclic aromatic hydrocarbons and form when muscle meat, including beef, pork, fish, and poultry, is cooked. These substances are known to cause cancer in animals; in humans, the association is still unclear. Continuously turning meat over a high heat source can substantially reduce such formation. Precooking in the oven, using thinner cuts that requiring less cooking, and, in general, avoiding prolonged cooking times are also helpful.

Processed meats. Consumption of sausages, hot dogs, bacon, and lunch meats, which are usually processed with nitrates, is associated with higher colon cancer risk. Eat these foods only in moderation, and be sure to accompany them with plenty of fiber-filled fruits and veggies.

Toxic fish. Mercury is a nasty environmental toxin produced by coal-burning power plants. It progressively infiltrates our marine food supply through rain. Mercury, along with other toxic metals such as cadmium and lead, can also poison bodily enzyme systems, as well as the mitochondria. These metals can cause blood vessel damage and contribute to hypertension, arterial disease, and heart attacks, as well as developmental disorders in fetuses and young children.

The FDA urges fishermen to pay attention to local advisories on mercury in fish in streams, rivers, and lakes. But the agency also recommends that consumers avoid the fish highest in mercury: tilefish from the Gulf of Mexico, shark, swordfish, and king mackerel. White albacore should be limited to no more than six ounces a week.

Because fish contains important nutrients and healthy fats for fetuses and young children, choose it with diligence and strive for two or three servings a month. And select from among types lower in mercury, such as migratory salmon, sardines, and Atlantic halibut, cod, and haddock.

Sugar in all forms, including high fructose corn syrup. The heavenly discussion surrounding one major toxin—sugar—floored me. Excess sugar, as I tell everyone, is the foremost enemy of cardiovascular health because it generates chronic, immune-destroying inflammation in the body; promotes weight gain and diabetes; and accelerates the aging process.

Many scientific studies have unmasked the deadly effects of sugar on the heart and the rest of the body. Case in point: A groundbreaking study from the US Centers for Disease Control and Prevention concluded, for the first time on a national level, that such a high intake of sugar actually doubles the risk of *dying* from cardiovascular disease!

The researchers aren't just referring to the sugar you might drop into a cup of coffee or tea. Many people worsen the problem by also consuming large servings of carbohydrates throughout the day, such as sweets, bagels, snack foods, pasta, alcohol, and grain-heavy meals. A high-carbohydrate diet, compounded with sweet drinks and junk food, can easily burden your body with a potentially dangerous sugar load.

According to the study, if your sugar intake is roughly a quarter or more of your daily calories, you have twice the risk of a cardiovascular-related death as somebody whose intake is about 7 percent. At around a 19 percent intake, the risk is about 38 percent higher.

When it comes to sugar, less is more, so if no more than 5 percent of your total daily calorie intake is sugar, I'd approve. For example:

Average Daily Calories	Added Sugar Maximum
1,200	15 g
1,500	19 g
1,800	22 g
2,000	25 g
2,200	27 g
2,400	30 g

Please note: I'm talking about "added sugar"—the kind you find in food, not the natural sugar in foods like fruits and vegetables.

This study also confirmed the danger of overconsumption of sugar-sweetened beverages, noting that seven servings a week—the equivalent of one 12-ounce can of soda a day—is specifically linked to risk of death from heart disease. This finding isn't surprising, since a common lifestyle choice for many people is to consume sweetened drinks like sodas, energy drinks, and sports drinks—the top offenders in terms of items with the most added sugar.

I recall a doctor friend of mine who was experiencing cardiac arrhythmia—his heart was skipping beats. When we talked about his lifestyle, it became clear that he was overindulging in sugar and alcohol (a major source of sugar). Luckily, I was able to set him straight and get him off the sugar, and his heart problem resolved.

I remember thinking, however, that if a doctor doesn't get the dangers of excessive sugar consumption, what about the public at large? Well, the public obviously doesn't get it. People are too fixated on the cholesterol-and-fat nonsense. So cholesterol isn't the bad guy in heart health that most people think it is? No, not at all, and I've been emphasizing this for more than 20 years. Cholesterol is, in fact, a natural substance the body produces to convert sunlight to vitamin D and to make sex hormones; vital, semipermeable membranes for your trillions of cells; and bile salts for digestion. Even your brain makes cholesterol and uses it to build connections between the neurons that facilitate learning and memory. Life can't go on without cholesterol.

Over the years, I discovered that cholesterol-lowering drugs are unnecessary for most people, way overprescribed, and not as safe as people think. The side effects are many—headaches, insomnia, digestive problems, muscle aches, skin rashes, weakness, and fatigue—and, unfortunately, often dismissed by doctors when patients complain.

I do believe, however, that it is smart medicine to give cholesterol-lowering drugs to men with known coronary artery disease who are under age 75. The research, as well as my own clinical experience, has shown the efficacy in this population to be certain enough to risk the side effects.

But I don't generally believe in treating cholesterol numbers alone. For some patients who want to lower their cholesterol, I prefer and recommend citrus bergamot (an extract from a bitter, fragrant citrus fruit called bergamot), fast-acting niacin, and omega-3 essential fatty acids. Cooking with extra virgin olive oil will also increase "good" high-density lipoprotein (HDL) cholesterol as well as support a fluffier "bad" low-density lipoprotein (LDL) particle, rendering it less inflammatory.

But back to that sweet destroyer of heart health: Sugar intake has an association with cancer, as well. Cancer cells have a different metabolism than normal cells and thrive on sugar. This understanding was first brought to public attention by the research of Nobel Laureate Otto Warburg in the 1920s.

Tommy's Teacher revealed that sugar affects white blood cell count. This is medically true, and I'll amplify: Excess sugar definitely suppresses the immune system, of which white blood cells are a part. Refined sugar inhibits the ability of white blood cells to fight off viruses and dangerous bacteria.

What's more, sugar accelerates aging of the body through a process called glycation, in which sugar compounds bond with collagen, proteins that make up the body's structural connective tissues, such as ligaments, tendons, and skin. Loss of collagen is a cause of wrinkles, which is a cosmetic change but can be enough to motivate many people to change their lifestyle. But more seriously, it also leads to rigid, less functional blood vessels and organs and weakened musculature.

Tommy's Teacher told him to drop refined sugars altogether. This is wonderful health advice for the reasons I mentioned above. So how do you do that?

Begin by cutting out one serving of food containing sugar per day. This might include the obvious: ditching the sugar in your coffee or tea, that morning doughnut, that daily hamburger bun or plate of pasta, dinner rolls from the restaurant bread basket, or a daily can of soda, to name just a few items. Eventually you'll want to get rid of other foods that contain refined sugar. After about 10 days of not eating the stuff, you'll find that you stop craving sugary foods and sweet things will even taste sickening.

Read food labels. Refined sugar has dozens of aliases, including sucrose, dextrose, fructose, and high fructose corn syrup and is hidden in many surprising foods, such as frozen vegetables, dry cereals, condiments, and marinara sauce. To be safe, try to keep as much as possible any foods that come in packages out of your house.

Cut back on artificial sweeteners, as well as the more "natural" ones. These days, many sweeteners are touted as "healthier" options. Don't buy into the hype. No matter what outfit it has on— raw sugar, agave, or molasses (and even maple syrup or honey, which offer some nutritional benefits)—if it is sweet; composed of sucrose, glucose, or fructose; and raises blood sugar, it needs to be used in strict moderation.

As for artificial sweeteners, they can be even worse for you. Chemical sugar substitutes like aspartame, sucralose, or saccharin have rap sheets riddled with controversy over their effects on the body, which include headaches, weight gain, and even the possible development of diabetes, heart disease, or cancer. If you've got to feed a sweet tooth, opt for very small amounts of honey, maple syrup, or the natural sweetener stevia.

In addition to the foods and substances I listed above, avoid these foods, too.

1. **Dill pickles and olives.** Both are loaded with sodium.

2. **Hot dogs.** These contain too much salt, as well as nitrates and nitrites, both linked to cancer.

3. **Deep-fried foods.** They're loaded with contaminated oils.

4. **Flame-broiled fast-food chicken.** This is packed with way too much sodium.

5. **White flour products.** They spike your blood sugar.

6. **Veal.** This is a highly inflammatory meat.

7. **Dehydrated soups.** They contain way too much sodium.

8. **Sherbet.** A lot of people believe sherbet is healthier than regular ice cream. Not necessarily. If you must eat frozen desserts every so often, go with a gourmet ice cream (one not containing high fructose corn syrup) over sherbet. Sherbet is pure sugar, whereas ice cream contains some fat and protein, both of which will help assuage sugar and insulin spikes.

Nutritionally, another way to honor the Body Temple is to steer clear of fast foods. A 2015 investigation by British researchers found that the more fast-food outlets in a neighborhood, the greater the risk of diabetes and obesity among the nearby residents. The findings, published in the journal *Public Health Nutrition*, were based on three public diabetes screenings in the general population as well as in "socially deprived areas." There were a higher number of fast-food outlets in nonwhite ethnic areas and poorer neighborhoods.

A US study in the same journal reported that customers who frequented urban corner convenience stores, also known as bodegas, spent on average $3 per visit. Their most common purchases were sodas, chips, prepared food, pastries, and candy. Regular soda was the most popular beverage purchase.

Corner store purchases averaged 66 grams of sugar—an amount equal to about 16 teaspoons of sugar. The average American consumes about 22 teaspoons a day, three times what's recommended. The study was based on nearly 10,000 surveys at 192 stores in a low-income area in Philadelphia.

Sadly, we live in a junk food society. Food choices make a big difference in how healthy and heavy we are and even how our brain functions. It is unfortunate that the worst foods are widely advertised and thus in high demand. No wonder there is rampant chronic unwellness, such as adult-onset diabetes, that is now increasing at an alarming rate and, most startling of all, affecting significant numbers of children. Diabetes is a gateway to cardiovascular, kidney, and nerve diseases.

With fast foods and other bad foods out of the way, what is the healthiest way to eat?

I've advised my patients to choose lean proteins based on wild-caught fish, free-range chicken, pork, beef, or buffalo, organic dairy products and eggs, and non-GMO soy products like tofu, edamame, or tempeh. Fish, a staple of both Mediterranean and Asian diets, is also full of anti-inflammatory omega-3 essential fatty acids. Eating organic or wild-caught sources of protein helps you avoid pesticides, antibiotic residues, and artificial hormones permitted in conventional food production.

Fats are important, too. Our brains, for example, are comprised of more than 60 percent fat. Fats help our bodies absorb nutrients like fat-soluble vitamins A, D, E, and K, as well as protective antioxidant compounds called carotenoids. Fats can actually help us lose weight when eaten in moderation.

It's not whether we should eat fats but which kinds of fats we should eat. Many doctors credit the enhanced longevity and health patterns of Mediterranean people to the large quantity of olive oil in their diets. Studies show that olive oil, primarily a monounsaturated fat, lowers risk of heart disease and breast, skin, and colon cancers. Research also indicates benefits for arthritis and diabetes. Olive oil contains phenols and squalene, an immunoprotective factor, as well as potent antioxidants that help support healthy immune function and blood pressure. I have always thought olive oil to be the secret sauce of the Mediterranean diet because of its multiple heart-supporting properties. Heat damages its health-enhancing compounds, so uncooked olive oil is best.

Avocados are another great source of healthy fat, and specifically alpha-linolenic acid (ALA), an essential fatty acid (EFA). They provide valuable antioxidant and anti-inflammatory protection, in part from a rich concentration of glutathione, an anticarcinogenic antioxidant. Other important qualities of avocados: lots of minerals, vitamin E, folic acid, vitamin B_6, pantothenic acid (a B vitamin), and the ability to help the body absorb vital carotenoid nutrients such as lycopene and beta-carotene. And, as I mentioned earlier, omega-3 fats, found in fish and flaxseed, have an impressive resume of health benefits.

As for carbohydrates, I suggest sticking to:

- Slow-burning, low-sugar vegetables such as asparagus, broccoli, kale, Brussels sprouts, and spinach

- Legumes such as lentils, soybeans, and chickpeas

- Onions and garlic

- Fruits such as cherries, peaches, plums, strawberries, blueberries, apricots, pears, kiwifruit, and apples (melons and grapes are suitable, but they contain more sugar)

Buy mostly organic fruits and vegetables, too, and eat five to nine servings daily. It's true that these foods, particularly fruits, contain sugar. It is natural sugar, however, blended in with the highly nutritious phytochemicals, antioxidants, and fiber found abundantly in plant foods. Most fruits will not adversely affect blood sugar unless you have diabetes. Patients with such sugar concerns must use some discernment and limit higher-sugar fruits, such as watermelon, honeydew melon, mango, and papaya.

The beauty of buying organic foods is that they have a high vibration—a property that was discovered more than 70 years ago by Dr. Royal Raymond Rife, whom Tommy mentioned earlier in this book. As noted in the book *Whole Health*, by Mark Mincolla, PhD, Rife became well-known for showing that different diseases have different frequencies and that certain frequencies can prevent disease, while others would destroy disease. (Frequency is the number of vibration cycles per second and expressed in hertz.)

Using a technology he developed, Rife determined that fresh, organic foods vibrated at an average of 20 to 30 hertz, higher than processed or dried foods. So if you want to raise your own vibration and improve your diet and health, eat high-vibration foods. When you do so, you can improve your immunity, cardiovascular system, digestion, and, indeed, your overall health.

Not only can you choose high-vibration foods, you can choose anti-inflammatory foods, many of which are also high vibration. Inflammation is essential for healing, but it can get out of hand. Chronic inflammation occurs when the body is repeatedly exposed to foreign substances (antigens), such as sugar, artificial colorings and ingredients, allergenic foods, environmental toxins and pollution, or the presence of an autoimmune disease, whereby a part of the body itself becomes the antigen and is attacked by the immune system.

Anti-inflammatory foods help fight chronic inflammation. These foods include organic fresh fruits and vegetables (such as kiwifruit, cherries, broccoli, and kale), wild-caught fish, and legumes—all of which supply our bodies with necessary nutrients and fiber without causing inflammation. Fruits and vegetables also contain valuable nutrients and antioxidants that fight inflammatory free-radical damage. These foods help the body process and eliminate toxins through healthy organ and removal mechanisms and give us the building blocks for robust bodies and the raw materials to generate the energy that keeps our trillions of cells functioning optimally.

At the same time, you'll want to avoid inflammatory foods. Generally, processed foods or any foods containing refined sugars that your body digests quickly are inflammatory (cookies, candies, sodas, white bread, pastas, etc.). Processed foods also tend to be loaded with trans fats, which contain inflammatory chemicals that increase shelf life.

I generally advise my patients to construct a daily diet in which about a fourth of their food comes from lean protein sources such as fish, poultry, pork (an excellent source of CoQ10), lean beef, bison, and lamb and vegetable sources like legumes. The remaining 75 percent of the diet should be split among healthy fats (such as olive oil, coconut oil, avocados, nuts, and seeds) and low-sugar, high-fiber foods such as greens and root vegetables—literally all types of veggies, as well as fresh fruits.

I am not a fan of whole grains because many of them are not only GMOs, but several cause an excessive insulin response. And some people are gluten sensitive. Three grains that are acceptable are amaranth, buckwheat, and quinoa.

Tommy's Teacher mentioned that a healthy digestive system helps eliminate toxins—also true. Honor your digestive system. One way to support your digestive function is by taking probiotics to help populate your gut with health-promoting bacteria. Probiotics help support not only your digestion but also your immune system. You can take them in capsule or powder form and/or eat lots of fermented foods such as yogurt, unpasteurized kimchi, sauerkraut, and miso.

Aim for at least 2 billion CFU (colony forming units) a day of *Lactobacillus* and *Bifidobacterium* species.

Be sure to stay well hydrated. Lack of water contributes to inflammation, moodiness, digestive problems, colon cancer, and possibly other cancers. Good hydration, on the other hand, has a cleansing effect on your lungs, kidneys, colon, and skin. Metabolism—the body's food-to-fuel process—is charged up by adequate water intake, too. Drink half of your weight in ounces of water daily to get what you need. Whenever you experience sugar cravings, immediately drink some water, which will help stifle the sugar urge. When possible, choose water in glass over plastic bottles to limit your exposure to phthalate, a harmful toxin found in plastic water bottles, as previously discussed.

Finally, get into the habit of offering a prayer of thanks for the bounty and blessings of your meals. Mealtime prayer allows us to slow down and not gulp down our foods, a habit that can lead to indigestion and poor absorption of nutrients. Prayer also encourages us to start our meals in a state of gratitude for what's going right in our lives.

Nutritional habits all add up—for better or for worse. Every new day is the perfect day to make the best choices you can to support your temple.

Applying the Revelation of
THE BODY TEMPLE

Commit to treating your body as the temple that it is. It is one of the most precious gifts you ever receive, a divine creation that deserves to be cherished and used fully. We expect a lot from our bodies every day, so let's affirm their right to expect healthy nourishment from us. Make a commitment to eat well, hydrate, and follow guidelines of good nutrition. Then consider the following action steps.

- At each meal, I will eat the healthiest, freshest, most colorful foods, organically grown when possible. These include:

  - Blue/purple foods: beets, black beans, blackberries, black currants, blueberries, eggplant, plums, purple cabbage, and purple grapes

  - Green foods: artichokes, asparagus, avocados, broccoli, Brussels sprouts, celery, collards, cucumbers, green apples, green beans, green bell peppers, green cabbage, green grapes, kale, kiwifruit, lettuce, limes, mustard greens, okra, peas, spinach, watercress, and zucchini

  - Orange foods: apricots, cantaloupe, carrots, orange bell peppers, oranges, peaches, pumpkin, squash, and sweet potatoes

  - Red foods: apples, cherries, cranberries, kidney beans, pink grapefruit, red beans, red bell peppers, red grapes, strawberries, tomatoes, and watermelon

  - Yellow foods: non-GMO corn, grapefruit, lemons, pears, and yellow bell peppers

- I will eat healthy proteins such as lean meat (for example, bison and chicken), nontoxic fish, and plant proteins such as beans and

Applying the Revelation of the Body Temple (continued)

legumes and cut back on my intake of processed carbohydrates such as breads and other baked goods. I will avoid toxic foods such as sugar and processed products that harm my body, and I will keep my body well hydrated. I will be mindful of how much I am eating and be more conscious of each bite so that I do not eat more than my body needs or wants, which can send me into poor health. I will eat to the point of just being comfortably full. Choosing well makes me feel well.

- I will live healthfully not only for myself but also for my loved ones so that they may be empowered to improve their health, too. When I fix meals for others, I will do so with gratitude, mindfulness, and a loving heart so that we can all live a better life. And I will give thanks for the gift of healthy food, for the Earth from which it grew, for the hands that prepared it, and to the Divine Being who provides all nourishment.

CHAPTER
8

THE REVELATION
of POSITIVITY

AS MY TEACHER FINISHES explaining the Body Temple to me, he transports us to the top of a magnificent snow-capped mountain, encircled by white, cottony clouds. Giant evergreens poke out from the snow. I reach down to touch it and am surprised to discover that it doesn't feel like snow at all but, rather, like the smoothest silk. I lie on my back in the snow and fan my arms and legs wildly, to create my very own snow angel. I feel so full of joy, happiness, and excitement. My Teacher smiles, clearly enjoying my childlike moment.

> *Men and women who grow up only to lose their childlike purity and joyfulness suffer needlessly in life. The key to happiness is simplicity. Enjoying the gift of life and every moment in it is like creating a new jewel for God's necklace. You do not have to be young to have joy. Every moment in life can be a jewel.*

Everyone has a pure nature, like a child's. This is impor-
tant, because children are more optimistic than adults. They
can quickly release anger and then get right back to happily
playing. Most children expect good things to happen to them.
They believe it and are willing to do things to manifest it.

There is a lesson here regarding the power of your thoughts.
They are the most powerful, creative tools in the universe. They
create emotions. Emotions create chemicals that destroy or
heal. Stay aware of your thoughts and feelings. A positive mind
cultivates positive results.

His teaching is the Revelation of Positivity.
My Teacher continues:

There are positive thoughts and negative thoughts. Just
like everything in the physical world, both have vibrations.
Good thoughts and words, like love, gratitude, and apprecia-
tion, create higher vibrations. If you are feeling happy and
thinking positive thoughts, you are giving out high vibrations
and creating health and healing. Bad thoughts, like put-
downs, unfair criticism, despair, pessimism, and anxiety, cre-
ate low vibrations.

As for health, if you constantly have thoughts of sickness or
disease, your body will convert those thoughts into physical
form. And remember what I said: All negative thoughts and
emotions create toxins on an emotional and physical level that
lower your vibration. Positive thinking produces a positive effect
on the body, mind, and spirit.

I can feel him looking deep inside me to see if I understand. I'm
a bit overwhelmed by all this information. In the past, I never
thought of myself as much of a positive thinker. I had good days and
I had bad days, ups and downs, and just went with the flow. I never
really paid a lot of attention to my thoughts.

As you stay here and learn by my side, you will come to understand the power of positivity. If people understood the impact of their thoughts on their lives, they would surely spend far more time cultivating positive thoughts. So make sure your thoughts are pure and peaceful and filled with unconditional love. This is how you create a positive reality.

Your thoughts are actions, too. They begin a chain of events, positive or negative, just as if they were physical actions. That is why it is so important to become aware of your thoughts and become a positive thinker.

Know, too, that every thought you and everyone else has is recorded here in Heaven, and you are responsible for them. I could show you where all your thoughts and the actions that resulted from them are stored, but that is unnecessary. Instead, understand this: Your thoughts are imprinted onto your spirit. They become part of you and help define you and the character you build and maintain. You are a collection of your thoughts and actions.

The power attached to our thoughts sounds so amazing: Our thoughts create our character, and our character influences the circumstances of our lives—health, happiness, our whole way of being in the world.

Still, I think how easy it is to lapse into negative thoughts. I remember after I got out of high school, I didn't have a chance to go to college. For a long time, I considered this a strike against me. I felt bad about myself, inferior to others with a college education. My biggest challenge back then was to develop a healthy dose of self-esteem. I finally took a serious look at myself and said, "Yes, you can be successful." After going to trade school to become a plumber, I ultimately built a thriving business and made a good living. So I've seen both sides of the mental coin: how negativity can hold you back and positivity can push you forward.

As I remember these things, my Teacher tells me about affirmations to kick out negativity.

> An *affirmation is a statement that helps you crystallize and align your specific intention with what God wants for you. Affirmations are very powerful tools that change thinking and, therefore, change reality. You will remember these words. They are being stored in your mind and in your heart:* "There will be no negativity in my life from this day forth. A positive attitude creates positive results."

I understand from this that although we can't control certain events in our lives, we can control our thoughts. I can react positively or negatively to the circumstances I find myself in. If I wake up in a bad mood, feeling stressed, worried, and anticipating a tough day, then generally I'll have that sort of day. If I'm positive, looking for something special in the day, I'll breed positive experiences. I bring into my life what I expect to find.

All of this knowledge is empowering. It makes me feel better about my life and the possibilities for my health. And it's knowledge accessible to anyone, college educated or not!

The Sinatra Prescription on Positivity

The power of positivity across every facet of life, including health, has never been in question. As a doctor and healer, I've always tried to impress on people that if they think well, their bodies work well. If someone is ill, no matter how seriously, I tell them that they must cultivate a belief that they will recover. You have the power to choose thoughts that enhance your health and uplift your spirit.

Tommy learned in Heaven that thoughts emit powerful vibrations (energy), which is exactly what Albert Einstein taught. He said that energy follows thought. So whatever you are thinking can become true, because thoughts are real, with their own energy field, and create your reality. Thoughts thus have a way of leading to what you expect, and those outcomes can be for you or against you, as we saw in the Revelation of Faithfulness.

When you strongly desire something positive and keep your focus on it, you will most likely get it. In 2005, I gave a talk on "healing the heart" to about 200 health-conscious senior citizens. As I looked out at them from the podium, they radiated health, vigor, and an absolutely contagious optimism, even though many had significant medical problems.

One gentleman stepped up to the microphone. He said he was 86; had aortic dysfunction, shortness of breath, and arrhythmia; and was somewhat hard of hearing. He'd had a quadruple bypass and a knee replacement.

"I want to make plans for the next 30 years," he said. "My cup is half full, and I want to make it fuller."

What an amazing spirit! That is the perfect healing attitude. Somebody else in his shoes might think their cup was half empty and draining, but not him nor the others in that room of positive thinkers.

When misfortune or disease strikes, we can make a conscious reaction—negative or positive. Some people develop a "poor me" attitude and turn into victims. They react to a situation by saying that "such and such has been done to me." In reality, nobody can make another person feel inadequate, unhappy, unloved, or guilty. These feelings and insecurities come from within and are drawn in from outside sources only when they confirm an inner belief. A positive response will only come when you begin to alter your own thoughts and attitudes about yourself and your situation.

Suppose you tell yourself, "My boss always makes me feel inadequate." Whenever you see your boss, your confidence shrinks and your self-doubt, anxiety, and discomfort skyrocket. In truth, it's not your boss who is robbing you of your confidence or competence. The boss is merely enhancing your already established feelings of inadequacy. Changing jobs won't alleviate the problem; it will only surface again at the next job until you find a way to internally control your self-evaluation. The best way to change the situation is to change your reaction to it: Develop a more positive attitude toward yourself and your capabilities. Start by simply thinking positive thoughts.

Behavioral research studies reveal that how we react to situations in our lives is extremely important as a variable in the nature of disease. Our character, adaptability, and responses to events may determine whether we get sick or not.

Many people see illness in terms of spiritual or emotional growth. Referring to their illnesses, patients have told me, "God placed it in my path so I will be more humble" or "to get out of a bad relationship" or "to change my bad habits." Those are the people who tend to recover most quickly.

Even if a devastating illness slaps us in the face, we have to find the blessing in the situation. I had a patient, Ross, who needed to undergo emergency bypass surgery. Afterward, he participated in our hospital cardiac rehabilitation program and weekly couples groups. He described how his attachment to his job had run—and ruined—his life. As a workaholic, he'd had no room for anything else. His heart had not been open to his family, friends, or even his own feelings. We explored further the reasons Ross had heart disease, because he did not fit the typical profile. Ross was tall and slim, did not smoke or drink, and ate a healthy diet. We determined that his problem was a thought pattern—largely thinking that he was desperately trapped in his job and there was no way out—that led to deadly stress.

Ultimately, Ross changed his thinking. He made the conscious decision that he was not going to die for his job. He looked deeper into his emotional and spiritual self. An early retirement package was offered, and Ross took it. He sold his house and moved to a small New England college town to be closer to his sons.

I tell this story to illustrate how if we find a positive message amid the negativity and make choices based on that discovery, our lives will unfold in a positive way.

I'm a perennial optimist, but this doesn't mean I'm a Pollyanna wearing a smiley face all the time. Nor do I deny the negative feelings that my patients with chronic diseases may experience. But I encourage them to do what they can to enhance their own positivity, because that, in turn, will help them be more successful in addressing the challenges they face with their health and with life in general. Even if you become seriously ill, try to stay positive. Positive intention is vital for healing. Negative thoughts are toxic to the body.

I can assure you, from observing thousands of patients, that positivity counts. You can choose to be depressed and live with the biochemistry that depression creates in your body or to be optimistic, find purpose in life, and live with the molecules that optimism creates. It's those molecules that help you recover and stay healthy.

In 2001, a study published in the *Journal of Personality and Social Psychology* gave strong confirmation to the power of a positive attitude. The study analyzed the medical histories and length of life of nearly 200 Catholic nuns who had completed handwritten autobiographies during the 1930s, when they were in their early twenties. "Positive emotional content in early-life autobiographies was strongly associated with longevity six decades later," after the nuns had retired from years of teaching school, the authors reported.

A careful examination of the writings for such key words such as *happy, joy, love, hopeful,* and *content* found that the nuns expressing more positive emotions lived as much as 10 years longer than those expressing fewer positive emotions. The findings concurred with other studies showing that people who rated more positive on personality tests seemed to live longer than those who were more pessimistic. People who are happier and more optimistic and laugh more have less disease. The researchers also discovered that early mental function could predict which individuals would show brain damage typical of Alzheimer's disease some 60 years later.

My most successful patients have always been people like those nuns, with resounding positive attitudes. Freedom from disease and better health clearly require "radical surgery" to remove old thought patterns. Positivity leads to productive changes in actions that, if repeated over time, solidify into good habits. And good habits create good health.

So how can we change destructive thought patterns? There are several ways.

Remember that everything is energy, including your thoughts. Whatever you dwell on most expands. Dwell on what makes you angry and your anger will expand. Dwell on the good in your life, as well as what you want from that life, and the goodness will expand and your desires will manifest themselves. Should negative thoughts sneak up on you—and they will—learn to view them as feedback about what you don't want. Once you have that insight, shift your attention to what you do want.

Retrain your brain toward positivity. Begin by challenging any negative thoughts. Is the thought true or rational? Is it helping or hurting you? When I'd ask patients if they could take responsibility for their health, I'd often hear "I can't": "I can't stop smoking," "I can't lose weight," "I can't eat healthy," "I can't exercise," "I can't change jobs," et cetera, et cetera.

Those are some of the most dangerous negative thoughts that can enter your mind, because they're not working for you, they're working against you. You must shut them down immediately and cancel out that sort of thinking, because you *can* do all those things and more. I suggest that you talk back to those thoughts in your mind, saying to yourself that they are untrue or silly and countering them with positive thoughts that begin with "I can."

Try this exercise: Take two minutes to write down 10 things you

feel positive about—your children, your values, your faith, your character. Researchers at the University of Chicago found that when people recorded their positive feelings, they had significantly less worry
and lower levels of harmful cortisol. And, incredibly, this exercise
raised their performance on tests of memory and critical skills by
10 to 15 percent. Refer to your list often so that your positive traits
become woven into the mental fabric of your being.

Start being more optimistic. Research shows that optimists are
not only happier, they're also healthier, live longer, and recover from
illnesses better than those with less cheery outlooks. Optimists inter-
pret events in a way that gives them hope to keep on trying. You
might say they know how to apply both the Revelation of Faithfulness and the Revelation of Positivity in their lives. Pessimists, on the
other hand, look at an event with a negative slant.

One study from Harvard reported that optimism and joy can protect your heart by actually lowering the risk of strokes and heart
attacks. The researchers had reviewed the outcomes of more than
two hundred previous studies and found that people with the most
optimistic attitudes had a 50 percent reduced risk of having a cardiac
event compared with those less optimistic.

One way to start each day on the right foot is to think about what
you are grateful for. But that doesn't mean just rattling off a list.
Really take the time to contemplate your feelings about each thing
and internalize how each positive feature makes your life better.

Also, as you encounter frustrations during the course of your day,
try to put a positive spin on them, a technique known as reframing,
to encourage an optimistic perspective. For example, if you don't feel
like going to work, be thankful that at least you have a job during this
time when many Americans don't have that "luxury."

If you failed at a task the day before, be grateful that you learned
a lesson and may have the chance to try again. If a relative has irri-
tated you, remember good times you have had together. Reminding
yourself of what you are grateful for will promote optimism and hope

even if your life has been difficult lately. You'll feel serene as opposed to agitated and depressed.

Laugh often. Much research shows that laughter, just as exercise does, produces a high tide of endorphins, feel-good brain chemicals that reduce pain and generate a sense of well-being. Laughter impacts your physiology in specific ways to bolster health and healing by lowering stress hormones, raising beneficial hormones, and boosting natural killer cells and immunity.

Think of your body as one big pharmacy that is manufacturing a countless array of chemical substances based on your emotions. For your own well-being, you need more chemicals based on humor than on stress. I've often told patients to watch comedies as a kind of laughter prescription to reduce stress. My favorites over the years have been the 1987 film *Planes, Trains and Automobiles*, with Steve Martin and John Candy, and the earlier *Pink Panther* films with Peter Sellers; you probably have your own favorites, and I encourage you to keep those DVDs handy!

My wife, Jan, a cardiac rehabilitation nurse for many years, used to encourage her patients to bring cartoons about cardiology topics to rehab sessions. The levity always helped elevate the mood of people who were burdened with anxiety over their health. When chronically stressed, we invite into our lives many different health problems: high blood pressure, heart disease, diabetes, digestive disorders, ulcers, addictions, headaches, insomnia, even cancers. On the other hand, people who handle stress constructively are healthier.

Find your own personal antidotes to stress. There are a lot of stress-busting methods from which to choose: Exercising. Finding a hobby. Dancing. Playing music. Engaging in or watching sports. Spending time with your kids or grandkids. Doing crossword puzzles. Knitting. Painting. They are all out there. My antidotes are walking, grounding, and doing yoga when I can join a class. Whenever possible, I get away from my many professional and business activities to pursue my favorite pastime: catch-and-release bonefishing. I basically disappear for a few weeks with my wife in a warm, sunny vacation spot and spend time wading and fishing on the flats. It's a moving meditation for me.

Another part of healthy stress management also involves physiological interventions through mind/body techniques like yoga, meditation, tai chi, and qigong. These practices, when followed routinely over the long term, lower the heightened sympathetic nervous system activity associated with emotional stress. Regularly practicing any of these methods helps to train the body and mind to adapt healthfully to stress through relaxation and breathing. Grounding, which I discussed previously, also shifts the nervous system in a healthier, more-balanced direction.

As Tommy's Teacher suggested, affirmations are excellent tools for reinforcing positivity and creating healing. Affirmations are words or whole sentences, spoken out loud or meditated upon in the mind. They create energy and have their own vibration. In 2004, the *Journal of Alternative and Complementary Medicine* published an article by Masaru Emoto, a Japanese researcher who set out to prove that the energy we give off through our thoughts, words, ideas, and music affects the molecular structure of water. He wrapped vials of water with pieces of paper on which were written either *love and thanks*, *devil*, or *you fool*. The water was then frozen. The water exposed to *love and thanks* formed beautiful ice crystals; the words *devil* and *you fool* produced no crystals at all.

In a similar way, repeating a positive word or phrase can alter a person's state of mind for the better, all due to the higher vibrations given off by positivity. Here are some affirmations to repeat.

"I have everything it takes to heal completely."

"The more I embrace positivity, the healthier I am."

"I'm healing every day."

"I'm healthy and strong, and my energy and vitality are increasing daily."

"I'm grateful for my life. I'm grateful that I'm healthy today at this moment."

Another strategy I recommend is to chant, using sounds such as *om, hrum, hum,* or *shum.* These are prolonged vowel sounds that create vibration within the body, so they help tune up our out-of-tune energies. Used in healing rituals for thousands of years, chants have been proven scientifically to increase mental alertness, relax the body and mind, improve breathing, reduce heart rate, improve blood pressure and circulation, and awaken parts of the brain and endocrine system that are tied to everything from immunity to emotional behavior.

You can also interrupt or work through negative thoughts by listening to soothing music or music with life-affirming lyrics (but no heavy metal—research shows it abnormally accelerates heart rate!). You'll discover that the right music can lift you up and bolster a more positive mind-set. In turn, a more positive mood can help you cope better with negative emotions and circumstances, allow you to problem solve, and enable you to take action for positive results. So let music into your life.

Remember: Always choose your thoughts carefully. You have the power to control them. You can bring whatever you want into your life. It all comes down to positivity.

Applying the Revelation of POSITIVITY

We've presented many ways to build a foundation of positivity in your life. It's something that takes daily practice. Here are some commitment steps to help you get started.

- I will start each day in a few moments of stillness. My attitude determines what each day becomes, so during this quiet time, I will center my thoughts on positivity—what I want to accomplish, what I feel grateful for, and the goodness I intend to experience today. If negative thoughts arise, I will listen to them, but I will question them: *Is this really the truth? Do I know this to be what is really true?* I will relax amid bad thoughts and simply release them, like balloons into the sky. I know that negative thoughts will dissolve on their own, and positive ones will come in their place.

- I will select at least three health-and-healing affirmations to repeat this week and three more next week. I will attach them to my mirror, refrigerator, or office wall—anywhere I can see them—as reminders of the transformative power of positivity. I will explore and practice other tools such as chanting, singing hymns, or listening to music to get rid of negative mind clutter. Any one of these will produce a calm and relaxing effect that will eliminate any negative energy within me.

- I will make a written list of the good things that I have in life and the positive elements of my health. I will also list the things I want in my life, not focus on what I don't want or have. If I want better health, then I'll focus on living a healthy life and take action to do so. If I want to feel more connected, then I will

Applying the Revelation of Positivity (continued)

focus on forming loving relationships rather than on my feelings of loneliness and isolation. I will add or subtract from these lists as needed. I know that my life will head in the direction I'm facing. The more I face and focus on the positive, the sooner I'll see positive results.

CHAPTER
9

THE REVELATION
of SELF-LOVE

AS MY TEACHER AND I continue to travel through the magnificence of this place, I see a woman with beautiful wings on her back, obviously an angel. She is tending a garden, not with water or fertilizer, but with love that I feel emanating from her. She extends her arms, sending out love and light to the plants. As the light reaches the flowers, their colors intensify like the brightest rainbow I've ever seen. The grass beyond the garden is a vivid green, perfectly manicured, and every blade stands tall and strong. Nothing on Earth can compare to the vibrancy of the plants here.

Observing my admiration for the garden, my Teacher tells me that like everything in Heaven, the grass vibrates unconditional love. I feel it flowing even from me. I am whole, as if nothing is missing inside me. This love is all-encompassing, free of judgment or negativity.

How is this kind of love possible?

The answer, my Teacher reveals to me, begins with self-love—that we honor and love ourselves unconditionally. This is the Revelation of Self-Love.

> *To be self-loving is the foundation of divine love. Divine love flows eternally and unconditionally between God and all living beings and never wavers. But for you to truly perceive and feel divine love, there must be a foundation of self-love in your life.*
>
> *With this foundation, you can also love others unconditionally, as God loves you. You will be able to love without fear and without wanting.*
>
> *Self-love also activates the Divine Spark within you. You will become love, and you will find your life filled with miracles and possibilities. So love yourself first—without ego—and you will be complete within.*

I'm confused at first when I hear this revelation. I recall my Sunday school lessons in the past. Aren't we supposed to love our neighbors as we love ourselves? I thought that was taught in just about every house of worship.

> *Yes, it is right to be thoughtful and caring to others. That is important. But those acts of kindness do not preclude loving yourself. They are not mutually exclusive.*

I guess many people focus only on the first part—"love our neighbors"—and neglect the "as we love ourselves" part. Still, *self-love*—it sounds so selfish and egocentric to me.

My Teacher smiles as he answers.

> *Yes, so many people get "ego" and "self-love" confused. Let us examine ego. You have a phrase on Earth that translates ego rather well: "edging God out." When a person has ego, their opinions and their thoughts are what they consider to be the*

truth, and this attitude pushes divine guidance and direction out of the picture. So do not confuse ego with self-love for they are not the same.

Ego is the aspect of character that needs to be satisfied. Those who define themselves by and attach identity to what they possess—that is, their earthly accomplishments—and those who require recognition and applause at every turn are filled with ego. Ego has no place in spiritual life. As you grow spiritually, you will learn that it is the surrender of ego that is the true, first step to enlightenment. When your personal concerns expand to include the safety and welfare of all living things and when the interconnectedness of everything is recognized, honored, and cherished, then enlightenment is possible.

My Teacher then elaborates on something that, to me, was profound.

Ego and fear are the twin forces of human destruction. If you look back on all of human history, you can trace every negative action to ego, to fear, or to both. This includes every act against humanity, every war, and every act of hatred, revenge, or anger.

Listening to all this, my head is spinning with ideas and knowledge, but I'm no longer overwhelmed. I feel fuller and more "in the know" about how things really are.

All the bad stuff humans have ever done to each other can be traced back to ego and fear. It's unbelievable when you think about it! War, holocaust, ethnic cleansing, slavery, terrorism, religious persecution. It's all there, and it can all be connected back to ego and fear. It's us doing it to us! These lessons make so much sense. As I digest all this new information, I'm asking myself so many questions.

How could I have gotten it so wrong so much of the time?

How could we all get it so wrong?

Why do we keep goofing up? Ruining the planet, hurting each other? Taking over, pushing each other around?

In this instant, I recall a time when my own ego had grown out of proportion, to my own detriment. My plumbing business had become very successful. We were hired for every job we bid on. There was no stopping us. But as the business grew, so did my ego. I got complacent and sat back, saying, "I've got my way of bidding jobs, and it's working. I know exactly what I'm doing, and I don't need to do anymore." In other words, I wasn't going at it with the energy and heart I had before.

One time we lost a big job—we were underbid, something that had not happened in years. To say I was shocked would be an understatement. I couldn't believe it! But I knew I had become careless with regard to the bidding process, negotiations, and customer relations in general. I realized I had stopped thinking about the work and relationship that every single client and prospective client deserved from me. That was the last time I let my ego and pride get in the way of good business practices.

Ego and fear become unnecessary in your life after you have mastered self-love. It then helps you experience God's love, which never wavers. When self-love is not present, you feel separated from God. But with self-love and God's love, you experience no wanting, no lack. His love is eternal and all-encompassing.

One way to engender self-love is through forgiveness. Learning to forgive others as well as yourself helps you integrate life lessons in ways that grow your spirit.

Forgiveness is a concept that seems simple enough. You are asked to forgive those who trespass against you just as you seek forgiveness from God for your own transgressions. Why is this important? Can you truly forgive someone who has deeply wounded you, hurt you, and seems unrepentant in their actions?

You must, because forgiveness is at the core of soul growth. Without it, you could not grow past what has been done to you and what you, yourself, have done to others either mindfully or without intention.

Learning to forgive, that's so hard to do!

To understand the importance of forgiveness, you must remember that God created you as individuals, but you are responsible for each other. You are one member of the entire human family. And in this human family, no person is alone or without the need to forgive others and oneself. Each human being at some point in their spiritual evolution is imperfect in thought or deed. Therefore, you are urged to work together as a species in harmony and peace, and you can accomplish this only through forgiving and loving hearts.

I am guessing this means not holding on to grudges? I've had times in life that if I was wronged, I wanted to right it.

Think of a time like that. Through no fault of your own, someone deceived you or hurt you or treated you unkindly or unjustly. Now, think about how much time and energy you gave to the situation. Be honest with yourself as you calculate how much of your time was spent on thoughts of anger, and think how much better it would be to have that time back for more positive endeavors that would align your spirit more closely to the divine.

Holding grudges keeps you in bondage; forgiveness frees you. True forgiveness takes time and awareness. When you are wronged for whatever reason, whether it be ego or fear on the part of another, it is difficult sometimes to find love and compassion in your heart for the one who has hurt you. But forgiveness is always in your best interest, because if you become angry without resolution or feed the need for revenge or retaliation,

you are creating negativity. This negative energy can be over-
whelming and can consume your energy if it is allowed to fester
unchecked. Unresolved anger and resentment can build up over
time and lead to depression and a weakened immune system,
which allows disease and illness into your life.

Forgiveness seems a little like housecleaning. When dust and dirt
build up, you get rid of it. When there's too much stuff and clutter,
you toss it out or donate it. When you're thinking thoughts of revenge
and grievances, your mind is cluttered with things that are hurting
you and holding you back. Forgiveness is like one big, deep clean
that leads you to more joy, happiness, and self-love.

My Teacher is pleased that I am picking up on this important
aspect of self-love. He adds:

As you ask for forgiveness, grant it to those who need it
most. Be aware of the fact that whatever happens to you is part
of your own creation so that you can grow your spirit. Experi-
ence everything so that you may choose again and again to
walk the path of wisdom and love.

I see and feel so much love here. If everyone could be in Heaven
for just one minute and experience this love, they would want to live
in its flow forever.

It is a universal truth that the self must be loved. Self is
you, yourself. It is all of you. Flesh and bone are irrelevant.
Self and the soul are irrevocably intertwined. It is your essence.
To not love self is to not love God. He made you in His image
and likeness—whole, good, and loving, in all your glory and
possibility. When divine awareness is achieved through self-
love, not ego, your Divine Unconditional Love toward all
things grows within you. By loving yourself, you are honoring
God's gift of life.

I was made in the image of God, formed by a loving Creator who knows me and calls me by my name. I'm called to honor myself so that I can honor others. I'm not just my body. I have a mind, heart, and soul that need and deserve love and care as much as my body does.

This revelation comforts me, because I realize how much God loves me. Had I realized this on Earth, I think I might have taken better care of myself and been more forgiving.

Here in Heaven, I feel so close to the divine. My spiritual eyes have been opened, and I understand that to not love myself is to not love God and to be separated from Him. After all, He made me! Although we are unique in wonderfully individual ways, we are also radiant expressions of God himself—inherently whole and worthy and lovable. God's unconditional love is ours at every turn. Nothing can change that.

This knowledge inspires me to open my heart and forgive myself for whatever I wish had been different. It's time to love myself unconditionally.

The Sinatra Prescription on Self-Love

This revelation is so important to how we live our daily lives. We must all celebrate ourselves, promote ourselves, and work hard to fulfill our dreams and desires. In fact, if we don't affirm our value as human beings and make the most of our lives, it can be difficult to make personal changes, stay healthy, or care for others.

My approach with patients has always been to encourage them toward greater love. Love is good for us, whether it is self-love, romantic love, or love for family members, friends, pets, or our fellow human beings. Love is essentially a biochemical event in the brain.

Several years ago, researchers from Albert Einstein College of Medicine in the Bronx and the State University of New York analyzed about 2,500 brain images of 17 college students who were in the early throes of being in love. The students looked at pictures of their beloved, and then at pictures of acquaintances, while an MRI machine scanned their brains. (MRI technology can detect increases or decreases of blood flow in the brain, which reflect changes in brain activity.)

A map of active brain areas was computer generated, showing hot spots deep in the brain, in areas that are densely populated with cells involved in the production of dopamine, which is churned out when people desire or anticipate a reward. In this study, dopamine sites became extremely active when the students viewed their girlfriends or boyfriends but not when looking at acquaintances. The results suggest that love or being in love heightens chemical activity in the brain.

When you love or are in love, other chemicals besides dopamine are released: oxytocin and vasopressin (the bonding chemicals) and serotonin (a feel-good chemical). Collectively, they improve mental health, strengthen the immune system, and relieve pain. As you love, you have a higher vibration and attract more love into your life. You are filled with the natural positive energy that generates well-being, wholeness, vitality, and connection.

As Tommy's Teacher pointed out, self-love is the foundation of all love. Learning how to love yourself changes for the better you and the world you live in. When you love yourself, you can create healthy, balanced relationships with everyone in your life.

But where does such love come from? Does it originate from your mother or father? Is self-love a learned experience? The answers to these questions are not simple. But we do know that loving qualities, actions, energies, and even words are transmitted to children from their own parents.

My training in psychotherapy taught me that self-love develops and evolves from the moment we are born and begins to crystallize in childhood. Some childhood experiences that have been identified as influencing self-love are being praised versus being punitively criticized; being listened to versus being yelled at; being spoken to lovingly versus being discounted or mocked; getting positive attention and affection versus being ignored and having no warm contact.

A British study published in 2013 in the *Journal of the American Medical Association—Pediatrics* supports these points. Researchers combed through 18 databases, 6 websites, and supplementary material from January 1, 1960, to February 1, 2011, and found 22,669 abstracts having to do with confirmed neglect or emotional abuse by parents in children up to age six and whether that abuse affected them emotionally, behaviorally, and developmentally.

The conclusions of this review were startling. Indeed, children who had experienced this type of abuse showed negative self-esteem, anger, poor conduct, withdrawal, poor social interactions, lower intelligence, and other problems, particularly if their parents had been insensitive to their needs, hostile, critical, or disinterested in good parenting. This study is enlightening, though a very sad commentary on what bad parenting can do to kids.

Children who are respected as unique individuals, on the other hand, tend to develop greater self-love as they mature into adults. They are guided and supported while mastering developmental tasks appropriate to their age. The self that is the child's is cherished and nurtured. Unconditional love—which is based on acceptance of a person for who he or she is, not what he or she does—is a key ingredient in the development of self-love in a child.

Of course, not all children are brought up in an unconditionally loving environment. As I noted above, some are faced with cold, distant, critical parents, whose love is conditional. This kind of love carries a double message and narcissistic qualities; it is a love based on approval alone. Children who grow up under these conditions have a hard time loving themselves in adulthood.

Ellen, age 48, was a perfect example of someone with a deficit of self-love that began at a very young age. She was referred to me by her internist because of an irregular heartbeat that seemed to be getting worse.

My first meeting with Ellen was quite intriguing. As she discussed her cardiac sensations and irregular heartbeats, I could tell that she was in touch with a deep sadness. At age three, she suffered her first heartbreak when her father abandoned the family for no apparent reason. She grew up without the love of an important and loving parental influence, and consequently, she felt unlovable and lonely most of her life. In her twenties, she got married, but she suffered another heartbreak at age 36, when her husband left her. She remarried once again but, at 46, divorced her second husband.

From childhood on, Ellen had a strong distrust of men—and a strong dislike for herself. As it so often does, this lack of self-love manifested in unhealthy habits and a lack of self-care. She told me that she would rather let her body go and become overweight. Having been hurt by so many men, she had deliberately made herself sexually unattractive. She said, "Fat is unattractive, and it will never get you hurt." By creating excessive padding as armor, she felt that she was impenetrable. Ellen was also looking for love from other sources, primarily food. She eventually developed the closed heart that had locked her away from self-love—and all forms of love, really. Ellen was avoiding that which she wanted most in life.

Her body began to fall apart—with infections, colitis, and, eventually, heart disease. These physical problems were telling Ellen the truth about her fear, anxiety, and emotional scarring.

Ellen needed to love herself and establish a heart connection with a man. Ultimately, she began to work through her issues of abandonment, distrust, and sadness, as well as her attitudes toward her body. Only through healing those wounds and sealing them up with self-love did she eventually heal herself and, consequently, her heart.

Ellen's case is not unusual; it's universal. I have seen many patients whose lack of self-love leads to disease, and not just heart disease: obesity, liver disease, addiction, depression, and more—afflictions that can carry us to a premature death.

Because our life paths begin in childhood, what can we do to enhance self-love as adults? It is a tough but not wholly impossible feat. I think I have some solutions. While I was training to be a psychotherapist, I facilitated multiple Healing the Heart workshops for my patients with another MD and a Gestalt-trained psychotherapist. Group therapy was utilized to uncover suppressed childhood memories, which were being expressed in adult character and personality traits. The process of group therapy offered provocative exchanges in which participants could see their own "stuff" acted out in others, even when it was difficult to recognize their own issues themselves. In other words, oftentimes what we do not like in others mirrors something we fail to recognize in ourselves: something we may not wish to face or even consider about ourselves. Such guided insight can trigger an awareness that can create spontaneous healing.

To develop self-love, think about what Tommy's Teacher told him: Begin by forgiving yourself for the ways in which you have rejected or otherwise harmed yourself—by eating too much, drinking too much, becoming addicted to drugs or other vices, and so forth.

Simply stated, forgiveness means letting go of the past. The negative energy we hold from past insults attacks our spirituality and interrupts our ability to connect; becomes a barrier to faithfulness; and harms our physical bodies. When we can stop beating ourselves up over our failures and start honoring all our successes, we can achieve self-love. For some of us, this may require a long journey; however, there is a specific shortcut to the destination: Simply say to yourself, "I'm sorry," silently or aloud. Those are the most healing words we can express—to ourselves and to anyone who has wronged us. When we can say the words *I'm sorry*, the heart opens up to not only an emotional place but also a spiritual place. Forgiveness is, at its core, an act of self-love. Our whole lives undergo a magical change when we develop a forgiving heart.

There is enormous healing power in forgiveness, too. Let me give you an example from my own life. Many years ago, I was sued for medical malpractice. During the lawsuit, my back suddenly went out. I developed two bulging disks, and for several years afterward, I continued to suffer lower-back pain. The trial was literally breaking my back. Eventually, my back discomfort became so severe that I had trouble walking, sitting, and carrying out daily activities. I tried everything to get better—physical therapy, counseling, acupuncture, orthopedics; you name it, I tried it.

It wasn't until I sought the help of a spiritual therapist that my path to healing really began. She intuitively counseled me that in order to heal my back, I needed to grant forgiveness to the people who had wrongly sued me. We did a number of spiritual exercises and meditations, all aimed at helping me find a place in my heart to forgive unconditionally. One of these was to visualize the family who had "injured" me. She then asked that I honestly acknowledge to myself how much I had been hurt. She was clear that I was not to overdramatize the situation or place blame on anyone.

Following that exercise, she asked if I could find a place in my heart to forgive unconditionally. As she worked with me to forgive the family, she gently and supportively placed her hand on my back, focusing my energy to bring the forgiveness down to my lower spine.

Very soon after I started therapy, the discomfort in my back improved significantly. I could walk and participate in all my normal activities. A resentful back, like a resentful heart, creates a trapped negative energy field that can lead to disease or disability. Sometimes you need to forgive before you can heal.

Many years later, in 2005, I came across a scientific article published in the *Journal of Pain* about how forgiveness heals back pain. I could barely believe what I had found, but there it was in black-and-white: a study of 61 patients with chronic lower-back pain who were able to reverse it by adopting a forgiving attitude! The research revealed that patients who can't forgive others might be experiencing higher levels of back pain and psychological distress than those who can forgive. There is a definite relationship between forgiveness and back pain (and probably many other health conditions).

Self-love is about letting go of the emotions that do us harm and actively choosing modes of thought that lift us up. Forgiveness fosters humility, which opens the door to gratitude. Practicing gratitude helps us feel more appreciative of our own unique gifts and talents as blessings. If you have been buried or you have been distracted by too many other things in your life to take stock of your blessings, carve out some time to figure out what makes you special. Make a list of what you believe are your best qualities and put the list where you can see it every day, perhaps by your bed or on a mirror. Add to the list as you discover new things that you like and appreciate about yourself. Be proud of these qualities. Honor your life as a gift from God. When you honor yourself, you are honoring Him.

As the Revelation of Positivity teaches, we must change the way we think about ourselves; doing so helps build and reinforce self-love. Begin by monitoring and regulating your thoughts. Practice not saying or agreeing with any thoughts about yourself that you would not direct toward someone you love or respect. In other words, treat yourself as you would your best friend, and think about how you can actively develop qualities that you want in a friend, such as honesty, loyalty, warmth, and affection. Do not allow negativity to dictate your emotions or color your worldview. We know now that negative emotions not only blind you to the beauty of the world you live in but can actually lead to illness and disease.

Without feeling embarrassed or silly, look at yourself in the mirror each day and tell yourself, "I love you, unconditionally." Write a love letter to yourself about your life and all the blessings you enjoy. Although doing this might feel initially uncomfortable, your discomfort will eventually ebb as you begin to realize the truth and power in your own words.

Adopt other self-love practices. If you don't exercise, for example, start. This could be as simple as walking for a half hour daily, taking a dance class, or practicing yoga. Physical activity will help you understand self-love not just as an idea but as an action.

When my patients exercised, whether it was walking, playing doubles tennis, or swimming, they felt more connected with their physical bodies and they looked forward to these activities, in other words, their self-esteem soared. They were loving themselves more. Exercise or any physical activity has physical, emotional, and spiritual benefits.

Not only does exercise keep you healthy and control your weight, but it also boosts your self-love as you feel better about your body and how it performs. Exercise also acts as a natural antidepressant. You don't need to be a marathoner to reap these benefits. You can obtain them through the simplest of movements, such as dancing, walking, or riding a bike.

You can also practice self-love by doing nice things to your physical body: getting enough sleep, indulging in a massage, changing your hairstyle, or getting a makeover. These activities may seem simple, but they are actions that reinforce how much you value yourself.

All of your relationships—including with God or your higher power—are affected by how you feel about yourself. Having a clear identity, maintaining healthy self-esteem and confidence, and knowing the gifts and talents that make you unique allow you to attract and create relationships that are balanced and whole.

These are what we all desire deep in our hearts, and it is human to long for them because such relationships are good for us. Statistics clearly prove that happily married people have a lower incidence of heart attacks than single or widowed persons. Widowed people tend to develop disease at an alarming rate, particularly soon after the loss of their loved ones. Divorced people are more vulnerable to illness and cardiovascular problems than married people. And living alone is a coronary risk factor.

Love heals—us and those to whom we give our love. It assures our connection to the world outside of ourselves. It affirms our role in the bigger picture—that what we say and do matters and that our contributions count. Loving ourselves, knowing we are loved, and opening our hearts to Divine Unconditional Love make our experience of life special. If we meet life with love, we will find love.

Applying the Revelation of
SELF-LOVE

What actions can you take to enhance self-love and self-esteem? The overarching answer is to find the positive force in a negative event or experience that may have hurt your feelings toward yourself, to laugh at yourself and not take everything so seriously, to communicate honestly and not internalize personal or work pressures, and to reach out and love, accepting in return the sincere affection of others. Keeping an open heart means being vulnerable and able to forgive yourself and others, over and over again. These are positive forces and emotions that build self-love and healing. Self-love is one of the best elements of preventive medicine we have today. Consider, too, taking the following steps.

- I will take a few minutes today to jot down a few things that I love about myself and note the special qualities that make me unique. Examples: My adventurous spirit. My love of animals. My hair. My sense of humor. My ability to sing, dance, write, or otherwise create. I'll develop gratitude for my God-given gifts and talents. Knowing that I have been blessed with such gifts is the right inspirational fuel I need for life.

- I will forgive myself for bad habits that in the past stood in the way of my happiness, health, and spiritual development. There is no one without flaws, but I relinquish the control that shame, fear, guilt, and regret have had on me. As I look in the mirror to express self-love every day, I will actively forgive myself and others and commit to treating myself gently and with respect.

- I will periodically ask myself if there are a few things I would change about myself. I understand that change can be good, and I will formulate realistic steps and strategies to make it happen, so I can move from where I am to a better place, emotionally and spiritually.

■ I will be part of a divine experience today by reading a sacred text, attending a worship service, praying, signing up for a spiritual retreat, or volunteering in a way that will have an impact on God's world. Through this experience, I will open my heart to unconditional love, the love that God has for every human being, and allow the gentle wind of this love to touch every aspect of my life. From now on, I choose to love myself, opening the way to love and honor others unconditionally, and experience God's love for me.

CHAPTER
10

THE REVELATION
of PURPOSE

I SIT WITH MY Teacher among glorious gardens, blanketed with flowers and plants of every color, and I think about the schools in Heaven where people learn how to become more enlightened. I think about the angels and how they all have different divine purposes. A burning question crosses my mind: On Earth, what is our purpose in life?

People have probably been asking this very question since shortly after life began. Some of us might be disappointed with how our lives have turned out so far. Some of us may be sick or in pain, searching for health and healing. Some of us may feel lost in a world of confused values and uncertain outcomes.

I decide to ask my Teacher for the answer to this universal question.

The answer is simple: You live to grow spiritually. The relationships that you form with God, with self, and with others provide you with opportunities to achieve spiritual growth and awareness. Relationships are wonderful vehicles for you to learn about yourself and to express and share the unique gifts and talents that God has given you. The divine purpose for all living beings, wherever they exist, is to become examples of Divine Unconditional Love. When you become this divine love, you vibrate at a higher rate.

How can I ever begin to fulfill such a divine purpose? My Teacher tells me to "live through my heart."

Your heart should lead you through life. It is through your heart that you can truly connect with your Creator and your divine self. Living through the heart keeps you fearless and ego-less and connected to all things divine. When the mind leads and the heart shuts down, a person is in danger of losing his or her way. True faith can elude the mind but never the heart. Living through the heart allows an individual to keep a high enough vibration to maintain optimal, vibrant good health.

As he speaks, I realize that the heart is the place where life finds its purpose. This is a huge epiphany to me, a moment of great understanding.

Before the accident, I didn't give a lot of thought to my purpose in life. I went to work. I went to church. I volunteered in my community. I prayed, but it was usually to ask for stuff, like a kid might tell Santa what he wanted for Christmas. I had a good life, but its course seemed bound by routine.

I never really listened to my heart or whether God was speaking to it. Now I feel I'm reaching a point where I need to listen to my heart more, be engaged with God, and hear what God wants for me. What God wants for me is what I want, too. Still, living through the heart in order to find my purpose seems like a tall order.

My Teacher reassures me that I don't have to be perfect, nor should I set that as a goal.

There is no such thing as perfection when you live in the physical world. Think of Earth as a school. You are there to learn lessons, to improve, and to grow. The path to growth is filled with bumps in the road, poor judgment, lack of self-esteem, imbalances, and lack of self-love. All these issues create difficult, unfulfilling relationships.

So, mistakes are part of learning?

Mistakes are not mistakes. Mistakes are lessons for self-improvement. They are part of the journey to self-love, self-awareness, forgiveness, and, ultimately, acceptance.

I feel relieved when I hear these words, and I understand how intimately all of these revelations are connected. I think about how many times in life I've blown it and how much energy I expended feeling guilty, ashamed, frustrated, or disappointed in myself. I know people who have given up on their whole lives and given up on their purpose because they made one mistake. What if we all understood that failure was not failure at all but simply an experience? What if we learned from those experiences rather than ran from them? How much more could we achieve?

Of course, mistakes happen, because we're all human beings. They also happen when we venture into the unknown. We have to take risks in order to accomplish something new, and sometimes those risks don't give us the results we hope for. The trick is to bounce back from mistakes and learn from them.

I like to read about people who have done just that, and the Bible and other spiritual texts are full of them. Just a partial list includes Abraham, Moses, Solomon, David, and Peter. Though they messed up at some point, and often in big ways, they not only recovered from their mistakes but also used them as tools of growth. If I learned anything from these stories, I learned that God does not turn His back on a person who has made a mistake.

Seeing mistakes differently, as vehicles for growth and signposts for renewed purpose in life, is important to taking on a variety of challenges. Our attitude toward our mistakes can even strengthen self-love.

My Teacher nods gently.

Yes, learning to love yourself and others and learning to forgive yourself and others are the keys to growing your spirit and increasing your divine awareness.

I'm still thinking about all of this and all the emotions and thoughts that have run through my mind while I was on Earth. I admit to myself that some of my thoughts and actions have been less than divine. I haven't always lived through my heart. I've been selfish. I've been unloving in some moments. I've been egotistical at times, and I've already admitted to being fearful.

I've tried to be faithful and truthful, but if I examine my past, I certainly haven't been perfect. Thinking about all that my Teacher is revealing to me, I realize there were so many things I could have done better.

Become an agent of change for the power of good. You need not wear a magical costume with a cape and mask to be a superhero. The superpower you have is the power of your own heart. Your heart gives you the ability to love and to grow your spirit. Therefore, you can achieve your own level of divinity, and then influence the people in your life and the world you live in. Every soul has the ability to increase its own divinity through the power of prayer, hope, love, truth, and faith.

Throughout life, each person must balance what is given

with what is taken; what energy is expended with what is con-
served; what resources are depleted with what is replenished.

If you are in service to others, energy that is expended in
helping humanity must be replenished through sleep, rest, and
self-loving activities that rebalance and restore the mind, body,
and spirit. If the gifts of love and service are given without a
solid foundation of balance, then ultimately, the mind, body,
and spirit will grow out of sync with each other. It is for this
reason that many nurses, doctors, healers, health care givers,
counselors, and therapists fall ill or are stricken with disease
themselves. Their actions have created an imbalance. Too
much has been depleted, too little restored, and the physical
body is sending a clear message to the mind and spirit that this
imbalance must be corrected.

By paying attention to balance, each person can lead a
full, generous life. By widely using what is given energetically
and then restoring personal balance, you can claim full power
without having to pay an unnecessary price.

I find myself relating to this message. I worked from morning to
night. When not on the job, I did volunteer work, feeding the homeless or raising money for my church. No wonder I used to feel so
drained all the time. I had been clueless about balance. I wondered
if there were ways to keep that balance more in the forefront of daily
life instead of only when things fell terribly out of whack.

So I ask: Is there a way to stay balanced in the face of everything?

Yes. The practices of prayer and meditation are two of the
most powerful ways to rebalance the mind, body, and spirit.
Prayer is not a series of requests. Prayer helps you communicate
with God. You may pray any way you wish. There is no right or
wrong way to pray. God hears all prayers.

As for meditation, achieving stillness is a very important tool in your life. When you are still, you can integrate the mind, body, and spirit. Meditating and focusing on your breath is a time-honored way to gain access to peace, tranquility, and stillness. It is best to set aside time each day to meditate and rebalance to allow for spiritual, emotional, mental, and physical health.

This revelation encourages me to look into my own heart and find meaning and balance. I realize that I must learn to tap into my unique gifts and talents to find my purpose in life and not spread myself too thin attempting to do everything at once. When I do that, I can accomplish my heart's desires, deepen my relationship with the divine, and find fulfillment in doing what I'm called to do.

The Sinatra Prescription on Purpose

This revelation hit me in a very personal way. At a very young age, I learned to listen to my own heart and find my purpose. When I was 10 years old, my mother became very ill, a very frightening experience for me. It all started when she developed glaucoma at age 38. In those days, glaucoma was treated with huge doses of corticosteroids, drugs that increase the risk of diabetes, and that's what she was prescribed. My mother already had a family history of diabetes; taking corticosteroids only worsened her chances of developing the disease.

And that is indeed what happened. Diabetes. It gradually stole her health, as it had done to her own mother.

Diabetes struck my mother hard. She became a very "brittle" diabetic, meaning that her blood sugar levels were at times impossible to control. Her swings vacillated precariously between extreme highs and rock-bottom lows. As a result, sometimes she would lose consciousness.

I remember as a fourth grader coming home to find my mother in "sugar shock" or even unconscious on the kitchen floor, a result of a bottoming blood sugar. I vividly recall the panic I felt as I'd shake her hard to wake her up. She'd arouse and ask for sugar. I would grab some orange juice. If I smelled acetone (a sweet, pungent-yet-chemical-like aroma of the breath), I scrambled to administer her insulin injection, just as she had taught me to do. To say I was afraid of losing her would be an understatement. I became terrified of arriving home to find her dead on the floor. In fact, whenever I heard a siren go off while I was at school, I thought it was for my mom a few blocks away.

Patricia Kelly Sinatra was as tough as she was beautiful, and she never complained, no matter what life threw at her. However, she did admit to one fear: going blind. She had watched her own mother gradually lose vision because of diabetes. Now the same thing was happening to my mother. I shudder to imagine the mental suffering she must have endured as her diabetes began to erode her eyesight.

As she aged, her complications of diabetes increased. Eventually, additional health issues surfaced. Osteoporosis and chronic pain slowly but steadily undermined her health and vitality. She developed cancers of the skin, breast, and colon. As her eyesight slipped away, she had to use the walls to guide her path.

One day, while visiting me in my new home, my mother misjudged the doorway to our cellar. She tumbled down the unfinished stairs onto the rock-hard concrete floor below, fracturing bones in her back, arm, and face. She was hospitalized for a long time. Sadly, the fractures around her one good eye caused an additional loss of vital peripheral vision. Eventually, my mother succumbed to cancer. I was in my fifties when that happened, and I was at her side to help her with her transition to the other side.

My boyhood experience of watching my parent struggle with a chronic debilitating illness made a huge impression on me. It shattered some of my illusions about how safe and secure the world really was. I learned all too early that life can be tenuous and cruel. Knowing how my mother suffered and struggled with chronic, debilitating illnesses was the foundation for my resolve—my purpose—to become a doctor. I repeatedly committed myself to helping others who, like my mother, endured and battled to maintain health and independence.

When someone has a life purpose—a motivating force—he or she has a powerful will to be healthy and is driven to live in order to fulfill that purpose. Possessing a greater purpose in life is associated with better health, greater energy, and lower mortality rates among older adults. A sense of purpose may also protect against the harmful effects of stress, including sudden death or cardiac arrest.

Paul "Bear" Bryant, the winningest coach in college football history, died of a massive heart attack in 1983 at the age of 70 shortly after his retirement. His abrupt demise was termed a sudden cardiac death.

A death like this occurs once every minute somewhere in the United States. It's the leading cause of death in the 20-to-64 age group and usually involves a heart attack that kills within an hour of the onset of symptoms.

Underneath these cold, hard statistics emerges an equally important factor in the sudden death syndrome: the powerful relationship between purpose and health. I didn't know Coach Bryant, but we all know people like him. When someone loses the motivating force in their lives—such as a spouse or career—he or she can also lose the will to live. Perhaps Bear Bryant's life purpose was coaching. Perhaps when this vital connection was broken, he experienced heartbreak, which can often lead to a variety of cardiovascular problems, including heart attack and stroke.

On a more personal level, I had a patient named Kevin, a 60-year-old newspaperman, who descended into a health crisis after losing his sense of purpose. An avid tennis player, Kevin was in terrific shape and could beat anyone. But due to his "old age," he was forced to retire from the newspaper. He felt considerable resentment and anger toward his employers. He even had dreams about being asked to come back to work, of his employers telling him that they'd made a terrible mistake in letting him leave. Although he accepted his retirement with dignity and did not outwardly show anger, his dreams reflected the truth; they were full of deep feelings of sadness and despair. The more I spoke with him, the more I understood that he missed the feeling of being needed. Kevin's purpose for living had been his job, and without it, he felt aimless and lost.

Because Kevin could not find a new job, he had deep, resentful feelings of anger and rage. The held-in explosive quality of those feelings resulted in an attack of ventricular arrhythmia (irregular heartbeat), leading to urgent hospitalization and treatment.

For men in particular, job loss can be devastating, emotionally and physically. Beyond treating the physical, I tried to get Kevin to consider it his "job" to get back to at least one or two of his passions— playing tennis, writing, or something else that he cared deeply about but hadn't made a priority while he was working as a newspaper-man. I was able to help him see that his resentment toward his for-mer employer was only holding him back and that he had to release this negative energy and toxic hostility in order to regain his pur-pose for living and ultimately heal. His heart started saying, "Play tennis." So Kevin got back in the game with renewed vigor and thus reclaimed his purpose. In the process, his heart opened up not only to an emotional place but also to a spiritual place, and he survived his heart disease.

By renewing his purpose, Kevin also strengthened his will to live—an extremely vital factor in health and healing. I've seen people who've been told by their doctors, "You have six months to live" (which, by the way, is the worst thing a physician can say!), and they go right to their deathbeds around that appointed time.

On the other hand, I've seen people respond entirely differently. They say, "Oh, no, I'm not going to die in six months. I've got this new grandchild, new relationship, new job—and I'm going to be around a long time." Those people live not just six more months but for many, many years!

World War II veterans are a good example, and I've had the pleasure of having many of them as patients after very serious heart attacks. Some of these men had a minimal chance of surviving but did so against all odds. I came to believe that this was because they had faced overwhelming combat situations, and their will to live was so huge. Survival itself was their purpose.

My Uncle Ed was one such veteran. Before he left for World War II, he fell deeply in love with a woman—my mother's sister. Then off he went to the war. He was in dangerously heavy combat for two years, bravely fighting but watching his friends die. He was then captured and made a POW in a German concentration camp. The Russian army marched in and took over the camp, and Ed became a prisoner of the Russians. Miraculously, he escaped. Numb and barely alive, he found his way to the Allied lines. How did he survive? Ed drew strength from his love for his sweetheart, whom he knew was waiting for him—a love that remained undiminished through the brutality of war and sustained him through all his trials. Love was his purpose, and it kept him alive.

I wish I could take the will to live and put it under a microscope, but I can't. I know, however, that a sense of purpose, a sense of determination, and a sense of joy over life's gifts produce a physical reaction that no doubt enables people to prolong their lives. This doesn't happen in every case, but that will to live is real, even though we can't measure it.

Tommy learned from his Teacher that the heart is the place where life finds its purpose. This is absolutely true. The heart is the king of the body; it holds your passion and purpose. The heart will not only tell you the truth, it will force you to see the truth. And if you don't listen to its message, you can become severely ill.

Think about your life: Are you holding on to distractions and unhappiness that prevent you from living a life filled with meaning and purpose? What is your heart telling you, and how well do you listen? How do you use your heart when making decisions and finding your life's purpose? This is one of those easier-said-than-done challenges!

There's a mental imaging exercise I use with people in my Healing the Heart workshops that can put you in touch with your heart on a physical and spiritual level. It works like this: Start by reclining comfortably on the floor on your back. Close your eyes and take a few deep breaths through your nose. Feel the breath going in and out. Do this for a few moments, until you're totally focused on your rhythmic breathing. This helps quiet your mind so you can listen to your heart. The mind loves to collect details, analyze, rationalize, and compare things. And often, your head will say "No" while your heart says "Why not?" You can't switch off thoughts, but you can move your focus away from what you are thinking and more toward what your heart wants to express.

Now try to visualize your heart. What does it look like as it beats steadily in your chest? See your heart as a living pump pushing its life-sustaining force throughout your body. Hear the gentle pulsations of your heartbeat.

Once you begin to feel the strength of its beating, give your heart a color—whatever color first leaps to mind. Ask yourself how much space this color occupies in your chest. Does it fill your chest cavity or take up just a small space within your heart? Does the color radiate outward to fill your body? Does it extend beyond the limits of your body? Can you see the color glowing all around you? Exhale and breathe into the color and feel its presence.

Next give the color a voice. Listen to that voice. Ask it what it wants to tell you. Is something not quite right? Or are you hearing that you're on the right track? Is your heart saying that you can do more with your life? Is it saying yes to something? Is it saying no? Is your heart telling you to pursue something that you love? What is the voice of your heart trying to express? If you can't hear it clearly at first, then ask the color inside your chest for the answers and listen for its message. After you've received it, tell it to your heart.

Now let all your mental images fade. Open your eyes slowly. Lie quietly on the floor until you feel that you want to get up.

This exercise is not about performance. It's about getting in touch with what your heart is saying. The process can be a very effective maneuver for discovering unconscious drives that are much more powerful than our conscious thoughts. For my patients who prayed, meditated, or did yoga or qigong (a Chinese practice that involves slow-moving martial arts), it was an easy exercise. For many of my patients who experienced fatigue, depression, or vital exhaustion, the process caused them to fall asleep.

If you don't "hear" anything the first time, don't worry. Try to repeat this exercise every day and eventually, you'll get results. It takes only 5 to 10 minutes of your time each day—not a huge investment when you are working on being true to who you are and what you want to accomplish in your life!

Purpose may signify different things to different people. For some, the pursuit of good health can be like a hobby—and a life purpose at the same time. It could be as simple as making sure your family is happy and feels your love. It could expand to a wider vision, such as contributing to social change or giving back to your community or, perhaps, the larger community of humankind. It could be more self-focused—perhaps doing well on the job, being creative, or staying engaged in something that is a good fit for your mind, body, skill, and talent. What's important is embracing your purpose fully and living for it daily, because it strengthens your health and may even lengthen your life.

Tommy's Teacher also spoke about maintaining balance in life. You have heard the divinely inspired phrase "balance in all things." That is a true statement. Getting out of balance is so easy, particularly when you are overworked or have your priorities misplaced. Some people can be so purposeful in life that they go overboard and sacrifice other endeavors for the sake of their life's mission.

I know this all too well. It was the 1980s. My practice was thriving and growing, as were my children. My life was filled with a lot of purpose and hard work. My future was bright.

Then, one day during those busy years, another life-altering experience happened. I could not resuscitate a young, hardworking, hard-driving father my own age. My heart was heavy as I looked down at that stretcher. I was overwhelmed by a sense of failure. Someone like me just died, and I couldn't save him. Sure, that comes with the turf of being a doctor, and one who is constantly put in lifesaving dramas, but it's always a painful moment when you realize that your best just isn't good enough.

An eerie thought crept into my mind. I had the realization that, working as hard as I was, I could very well be that person on the stretcher. Young but dead. I didn't want *that* to be me.

My realization prompted me to enroll in a Gestalt psychotherapy training program, and what an eye-opener that was! I now began to consistently observe the close connection between stress, overwork, and cardiac events in my own medical practice. Type A behavior traits include overworking, overachieving, time urgency, and wanting to win at all costs: basically, a life out of balance. That was me.

As I saw these personality patterns in others, I continued to see my own 35-year-old face looking back at me in the mirror as I shaved each morning. These ongoing realizations confirmed the old adage: "Physician, heal thyself!"

Should I fail to address my own level of stress and Type A struggle to do more in less time it really *could* be me on that stretcher next. To tell the truth though, even after I became aware of my own Type A behavior, it would take me many years of self-reflection to change it and restore balance to my own life.

Disease and illness emerge from a chaotic, fragmented imbalance among the energies of mind, body, and spirit. Consider high blood pressure, a problem affecting more than 70 million Americans. Although, for some people, the source is an overactive adrenal or thyroid gland, others may be overweight or have emotional toxicities.

Stress is always a factor, especially when it involves job or personal difficulties, financial trouble, a health crisis, or loss. Anger is the Achilles' heel for the cardiovascular system because it drives up blood pressure.

While some patients grapple with these physical and emotional factors, others may be disconnected from their spiritual selves as well. For instance, after treating people with hypertension for decades, I realized during the last few years of my cardiology practice that patients who "did not tell the truth" or live authentically seemed to have higher blood pressures. After publishing research on grounding and heart rate variability, I found it obvious that any lie or falsehood was a betrayal of the self that would be expressed as a surge in the autonomic nervous system and, thus, have a negative impact on cardiovascular health. It took me 40 years of medical practice to realize that a common problem in high blood pressure is an unbalanced disconnect of mind, body, and spirit.

Warning signs that you may be out of balance include higher blood pressure, an increased heart rate, muscle tension, shallow breathing, trembling, jaw grinding, racing thoughts, nervous habits, and tightness in the chest. These symptoms, if recognized and addressed, aren't likely to harm you. They are the body's way of telling you that you need to pay attention and make some changes. I've used the following questions in my practice to help patients achieve more balance in a situation.

What am I doing?

Why am I doing it?

What am I hoping to accomplish?

Is what I do making me happy?

Am I revolving my life around making someone else happy at great cost to myself?

What does the way I live my life cost me in terms of time, energy, and resources?

Is there another way that I can invest my resources that will be more efficient and produce the same or better results?

While it is lifesaving to have purpose in life, part of that purpose should be to live a balanced, vibrantly happy and healthy life. If you know you're out of balance, prayer and meditation (like the exercise I described above) can help, as Tommy's Teacher pointed out. I should add that there is a subtle difference between the two. In meditation, we quiet ourselves to access our inner healer or voice and listen to an answer. Some of us may even ask God to come to us in meditation. When we pray, we reach beyond ourselves to offer our prayers up to God.

The fact that Tommy's Teacher mentioned both practices, in the context of finding one's life purpose, both uplifted and fascinated me. Scientific studies, particularly on meditation, prove this divine message to be true. Yes, an ever-expanding body of research shows how meditation can be used effectively to help prevent illness, treat specific conditions, and restore health. But more recently, this technique has been drawing scientific attention for the role it plays in encouraging people to find meaning and purpose in their lives.

One example: In 2012, researchers in Japan conducted a study of 54 university students, who were divided into two groups: an experimental group, instructed to do a daily 10-minute Buddhist-based meditation at home, and a control group, which did not meditate. Through questionnaires, all the participants were assessed before and after the experiment to determine their sense of coherence (a view that recognizes the world as meaningful and predictable), self-esteem, and purpose in life. The experiment lasted one month.

By the end, there were marked differences between the two groups. The meditators showed significant increases across all three parameters, whereas the nonmeditators did not. The students who meditated had a greater sense of coherence, meaning that they felt their lives made sense and life challenges were worthy of commitment, even in light of stress or an out-of-balance lifestyle. Their self-esteem was stronger, and their life purpose was more clarified and focused. So, clearly, meditation can help you find direction in life—and offers a way for you to listen to your heart for answers and insight into your own life purpose.

I have practiced Transcendental Meditation (TM) since the 1970s, and although I'm not steadfastly regular, the practice has often helped get me through intense times in my action-packed life. Simple and enjoyable, TM is an Eastern practice that combines clearing your mind of all thoughts, practicing deep breathing, and chanting mantras to put yourself in a calm and relaxed yet focused state. Moreover, the late Maharishi Mahesh Yogi, who founded the TM program, put great emphasis on scientific research. Most of the research, in fact, confirming the many health benefits of meditation has been done by the TM organization. There have been more than six hundred studies to date published in scientific journals about the benefits of TM, lending credence to the technique's reputation as the Rolls-Royce of meditation.

One study that caught my attention reported that patients with heart disease who practice TM long term have almost a 50 percent lower incidence of heart attack, stroke, and death compared to nonmeditating patients. Another study indicated that TM reduced blood pressure, anxiety, depression, and anger among healthy college students at risk to develop hypertension.

There is definitely proof that prayer and meditation work on a number of levels for physical and psychological health. I think we all know that intuitively, without having to read so many facts and figures in scientific journals. I like to think of prayer and meditation the way I do electricity. I don't have to know how it works to trust that it will!

In addition to practicing meditation and offering prayers, plan ways to make time for things that are meaningful priorities for you—your dreams, your goals, and what makes you happy. Take back your life and stay focused on fulfilling every one of your priorities to the best of your ability. Learn to say no, setting a boundary with real feeling. This is a crucial step in achieving and maintaining balance. The ability to say no and stand by it is one of the hallmarks of a healthy, grounded, and balanced person.

Other actions that restore balance include elements of proper breathing, exercise, nutritional healing, grounding, the release of painful emotions, reopening the heart to love, and the development of meaningful connections—all of which are inherent in the heavenly revelations. The path to restoring balance is another opportunity to listen to your heart.

Living through your heart allows you to keep a high enough vibration to maintain the optimal health you need to accomplish everything you were put on Earth to do. Last but not least, living through the heart directs you to live for something big. Look into your own heart for the message it is bringing you and ponder it deeply. Ask yourself: "What do I most deeply desire?" That is what God desires for you, too.

Applying the Revelation of
PURPOSE

In essence, the heart is where everything comes together, helping you find your passion and purpose in life. Here are some practical commitment steps to help you apply this last revelation to your own life.

- I will live more fully through my heart by asking and answering some simple but very key questions, such as: What are my passions? What are the things I really love to do, and how can I find ways to do them more often? What activities seem to drain my energy or distract from what I really want to be doing in life? What choices am I making about my direction? What does my life say about my relationship with God and with people I may be influencing? Through pondering these issues, I will find a life that is beautiful and inspiring, one that reveals new horizons and possibilities for spiritual growth and good.

- Once I identify my purpose, I will take steps to fulfill it. This requires setting well-defined goals and strategies, with room for change. Should everyday problems or even crises occur, I'll be more prepared, because a purposeful life has inherent solutions. Life may still put up obstacles, but I know that even an obstacle has a purpose, inviting me to grow, showing me another way around it, or offering me a chance to be the person I was meant to be. At the same, I will strive for balance. I'll say no when requests are impractical or emotionally taxing. I'll let go of the need to control and do everything myself. Periodically, I'll look at my life objectively and assess my level of contentment with my accomplishments. Does my work still reflect my passion and purpose? If not, it's time for me to prioritize the elements that fulfill me emotionally and spiritually.

■ For 5 to 10 minutes daily, I'll take time for reflection through daily prayer or meditation, so I can hear what my heart is telling me. I will give credence to what my heart is saying and look for ways to act on it. On occasion, I may falter, but I don't have to be perfect. I will acknowledge that mistakes are really only lessons in disguise. I will learn from them, recognize the positive aspect of the situation, and move forward—because it's never too late to get it right. To achieve my dreams and make the impossible possible, I must believe in myself, and I must push myself. The energy that fuels my fire and the excitement each new day brings keep me going. My motivation comes from possessing my God-given purpose and the vision I have for my life.

CHAPTER
11

THE GREATEST
MOMENT

MY TEACHER HAS REVEALED so much to me. It's ironic, but I feel truly and completely alive for the first time! I finally understand how things really work and what is truly important.

I have no idea how long I have been here. There are no clocks in Heaven, and I can't seem to measure time at all. Time feels different, like it doesn't matter. There's no sense of urgency, no rush.

I'm still not sure if I am alive or dead, although I'm leaning toward dead, since I know that I'm in Heaven. I did see my father and my grandmother again, and they have been gone for years, so it stands to reason that my time on Earth is finished, too.

Before this moment, I felt deep down that if I asked the wrong question at the wrong moment, my whole incredible experience would abruptly end, and I would stop feeling this wonderful love and peace. I'm now sensing something has changed, and I feel free to ask some big questions to the man who has been accompanying me throughout this experience. He has been such a patient guide, and I can feel his great love. It is in every word, every look, and every gesture. He is encouraging me to ask him what is in my heart.

Courage and a boldness of spirit swell inside me. So, I begin.

I ask him, "Can you tell me now why I am here?"

My Teacher looks at me with the greatest love in his eyes and says words I will never forget.

> *You are here at the present time in your life to learn the true meaning of self-love, awareness, and faith and also how to heal the mind, body, and spirit.*

Who are you?

> *You know me as Jesus the Christ.*

Somehow, I knew this all along, but I waited for him to confirm what I believed: that this man is indeed Jesus, God's son. But I almost can't believe it—Jesus! This must certainly be the greatest moment of my life—to meet the Jesus of my Catholic upbringing! I cannot express how awestruck I am. I know I have been blessed beyond words.

Humbled deeply, I ask him with the utmost respect, "If you are Jesus, who is God?"

> *God is omnipresent in All That Is. God is the Creator and my Father, but he is also your Father and everyone else's Father. He lives in each of you as an aspect of himself.*

I don't understand what he is telling me about God, so I press further. I ask Jesus most humbly, "Can I see him? Can I see God?"

> *Yes, I will show you an aspect of God so that you can see him.*

Jesus then raises his right arm over his head. As he lifts his arm, a bright orange, yellow, white, and blue light appears. The light is the size of a baseball, and it is radiating absolute love and peace. It's not like any light I have ever seen here or anywhere. The light is alive and conscious and so filled with love. It is so bright that it is hard to look at it. I know deep inside of me that either I or the light is being modified in some way so that I can actually see it. The light is as bright as the sun, maybe brighter.

There are long, beautiful rays of light emanating from the center of this ball of light. Jesus moves his right hand down, and the ball of light moves with it, hovering over his hand but not quite touching it. Jesus's hand is now outstretched in front of me, and this ball of light hovers over his hand as I watch in amazement. Tears are streaming down my face, and I find that I am trembling from head to toe. Rays of light from this ball are rotating in all directions. The source of light in Jesus's hand is glowing and living. The beauty and power and love from this source of light cannot be described. There are no words that can fully capture this experience. I can only say that I know deep within myself that this is some wonderful, beautiful part of what is God. I fall to my knees in awe and gratitude.

The ball of light disappears. Jesus brings his hand over my head, and I am flooded with more love and warmth than I have ever felt, even deeper than what I have been feeling throughout this whole experience. Nothing can compare to this moment.

Jesus looks at me with the greatest love and explains:

> This is what God looks like in this moment as pure energy, but He can take any form. I chose to show you God in this way because you cannot be with Him fully yet. It is too much. This moment is enough. You have seen your Father in All That Is.

As I formulate my next question, my celestial surroundings suddenly change. I am pulled back into the tunnel of light, this time going headfirst, on my back, in reverse. I speed through streaks of light that are everywhere, still feeling totally at peace, the same way I felt before. Within moments, I find myself back in my physical body. It's like a jolt! I am alive! I am awake! I am lying in a hospital bed, and I am in the greatest pain and agony I have ever felt.

PART III

TRANSFORMED

CHAPTER
12

BACK DOWN TO
EARTH

"**How did I get** back here?" I wondered, terrified and confused. "I was just in Heaven."

Medical equipment clicked away. A tube was stuck into my mouth, an IV was jabbed into my swollen and bruised arm. The room spun around me. I heard a voice calling my name.

"Tommy," said a nurse in a very calm voice, "you've been in an accident. You're unable to breathe on your own because your lung has collapsed. You're on a respirator now. You've been in a coma for quite a while. Try not to move too much. You need to be still and let your body heal. You can't walk."

I was so disoriented. There was so much pain. The whole time I was in Heaven, I felt no pain at all. Now my chest hurt so badly that I couldn't even take a full breath. I looked down at my arms. They were so swollen that I couldn't see my fingers. I couldn't move my shoulders and neck. My legs ached, and I was cold all over. I was in a state of total fear.

The nurse had mentioned an accident. What accident? I didn't remember any accident. I didn't even know how I got here. Wasn't I just in Heaven? Had it all been a dream? It felt so real.

Deep down, something inside me confirmed that it was all real. But I wished I was back in Heaven. I thought I was going to stay there forever.

I am so disappointed!

I never dreamed I'd be back in my body. In Heaven, there was no pain, discomfort, or suffering. But in that hospital bed, I was enduring horrible pain. It felt new and foreign to me. Profoundly disappointed, I was overcome with an intense longing to be back with Jesus. My sadness at being back on Earth was just as painful as my broken body. I drifted off to sleep, hoping I'd be pulled back into the light tunnel again.

That wasn't to be.

The next day, the tube was taken out of my mouth to see if I could breathe on my own. My vocal cords and throat were so raw that I couldn't speak. Doctors and nurses advised me to not speak. That was okay by me. I'd already decided to keep what happened in Heaven to myself. I felt too vulnerable and confused to articulate what I had learned and experienced; it was all so much to process. Who would believe me, anyway?

My brother was at my bedside. Should I tell him I had seen Dad and Grandma? He'd probably think I'd had a crazy dream or was delusional because of all the drugs that had been pumping through my system. Although our family is Roman Catholic and we always attend church, I decided this news would be a stretch. I kept quiet.

My brother told me what happened: "You were run over by a car traveling approximately 40 miles an hour."

I nodded in understanding.

"You died twice last week from heart failure and had to be

shocked back to life. Your head was twice its normal size, but it's much less swollen now."

To me, it felt as big as a watermelon.

My brother rattled off my numerous injuries. Not only were my lungs bad, but I had nine fractured ribs, seven herniated disks, six fractured vertebrae, a fractured pelvis, a fractured skull, and a fractured hip. I got exhausted hearing all this. No wonder I was in agony. I drifted back to sleep, hoping to get back to Heaven and Jesus.

The more I heard about what had happened to me, I was surprised that I was alive at all, even in my banged-up condition. I knew inside that this was the point in my life at which I had to decide to change some things. My heart, mind, and spirit longed to get back to the place where there is no fear.

As more days in the hospital passed, the pain only got worse. All I wanted to do was sleep to keep the pain level down. I had suffered from asthma before the accident, and now it was aggravated by the collapsed lung. Breathing was hard.

I grew worried about the long-term consequences of the accident. Would I ever work again? Would I ever walk again? I prayed to Jesus to help me overcome my worries about becoming a burden to anyone. I asked him to help me overcome my disabilities, to take the pain out of my arms so that I could feed myself and eat and drink to regain strength, and to keep me strong against my enemy, which is fear. Mostly, I asked Jesus to love me here, like He did all the time we were together in Heaven.

Before falling asleep again, I thought more about all that Jesus had taught me while I was in Heaven. I understood that I must begin applying the lessons I learned.

After I woke up, I could swallow and felt a real improvement in my throat. It wasn't as raw, so I hoped I could eat some real food. My brother snuck me a sandwich. I started to eat, but it got stuck in my throat and I vomited. I tried again the next day, and that time I could keep the food down.

I was still in a lot of pain, but I managed to pray every single day.

I still couldn't stand up, so I asked Jesus to help me walk again. The lower back pain radiated down both my legs and was excruciating. The drugs didn't relieve this pain, and I asked the nurse to stop giving me morphine. I would rather tough it out than have this continual brain fog. I think the morphine was making me confused. It was hard to remember anything. I had absolutely no memory of the accident or being run over. The few months before the accident were gone, too. I didn't remember my old life.

My brain function and mental reasoning were definitely off. People were visiting me, but I forgot that they came and their names escaped me.

But nonetheless, I slowly began to make progress.

Finally, after being in the hospital for several weeks, I was told that I could go home. I couldn't wait to get some fresh air and see the sky again. I was excited to leave but also a bit scared. I hoped I'd be able to take care of myself.

The nurse said that she'd get me a wheelchair on the day of my departure, but I stubbornly insisted on leaving with a walker instead. My legs were still weak, and my muscles, inflamed. I was determined to make it on my own steam, though. I dragged my right shoulder against the hallway wall for support, to keep myself standing upright. As I moved forward, my left leg went out from under me. Hospital staffers rescued me, firmly yet gently seating me in the wheelchair. I tried the walker again, resting every 20 feet or so to prevent another fall. My gait was off due to the multiple unhealed fractures. I was afraid that if I got into that wheelchair, I might never get out of it. I had to learn to walk again. I had to!

I entered my apartment, and it felt really strange, almost foreign. I collapsed into my chair. I was so tired and depressed. All my time with Jesus and His beautiful teachings were flying out the window. I was afraid that this terrible pain would last indefinitely.

I didn't know if I'd be able to work again. Maybe never! How would I take care of my financial responsibilities? How would I pay for my rent, phone, insurance, medicine, and food? It was much easier being in Heaven with no fears and worries about this earthly stuff.

Time passed but the pain did not. I felt tired, mentally fatigued. Going to my multiple doctors' appointments gave me something to do, but it was an ordeal getting there and back home. Someone had to take me because I couldn't drive. I felt like a burden, despite reassurances from friends and family that I was not.

It would be 18 months before I could walk without a walker or cane. My legs would continue to feel weak for a long time after that. Gradually, I was able to feed myself. Headaches persisted for two years as a result of my skull being fractured.

To help with the pain, I began seeing a chiropractor daily, except on Sundays. Chiropractic work is a great way to get the body's energy flowing because it removes blockages from the chakras. During my sessions, I recalled some of what Jesus taught me about energy and vibrations. I concluded that, to recover, I would have to push my physical body and get more health conscious. Waiting to recover was not the answer. I would have to fight my way back to health with God's help. I wanted to stimulate my Vital Force to get healing to where there was inflammation in my body. I tried acupuncture to move energy to the meridians. Treatments twice a week really helped me.

I started to go to church more often in order to recapture the divine energy I felt in Heaven. The peace and tranquility in church were soothing and serene and helped me let go of fear.

I still indulged in little pity parties from time to time, but my faith in God and in what is truly important crystallized because of my experience. I drew on that faith now that I was back, though in a broken body.

Miracles at the Grotto

One day during my recovery, I woke up thinking about a place from my childhood: Our Lady of Lourdes Grotto at St. Lucy's Catholic Church, tucked deep within the Bronx. It is a shrine to the Virgin Mary, a replica of Our Lady of Lourdes in France, where many believe miracles have unfolded. Maybe my guardian angel whispered "the Bronx grotto" to me while I was sleeping. All I know is that I woke up one morning and had to visit it.

Since 1939, people from around the world have gone there to pray for healing from cancer and other scary diseases or for the rescue of loved ones from their deathbeds. There's a stream that runs beneath the statue of the Virgin Mary. Its coveted water originally came from a natural spring, but the spring dried up long ago, forcing the shrine to switch to tap water blessed by priests. People still believe it performs miracles, and they douse their heads in the water, rinse their faces, nudge their children and dogs under the flow, and fill baby bottles, flasks, water and juice bottles, and empty gallon milk jugs with water they take home to bless family, houses, and even cars.

When I was a kid, my parents regularly took me to the grotto. I was born virtually blind in one eye, and they hoped that I might receive miraculous healing for my impaired eyesight. I loved going there. It was a special place that filled me with faith, and I was always inspired when I visited.

Now, as an adult in poor physical health, I knew I had to go back. My hope was that the grotto would bring back the feeling I had when I was with Jesus. So I went to visit His mother, Mary.

I started going once a week for an hour. I had to be driven, so I couldn't just go anytime I wanted. I would watch as the people lined up, patiently waiting their turn to fill their containers with the blessed water. Often, people dressed in full business attire would come up the steps and dunk themselves under the water, letting it pour over their heads and their clothes until they were completely soaked. They would emerge wet and filled with joy, shouting out their thanks to Heaven.

The grotto has the highest vibration of any place I've experienced since returning from Heaven. The people praying there feel it, too. The air is filled with hope and possibility. Praying there week after week lifted my sadness at being back in my physical body. I felt connected again to all that was holy. I was filled with true faith once more, and finally, I was truly happy to be alive!

During one of my visits, a tiny older woman wearing a slightly tattered coat approached me and held out her right hand. "Could you be so kind as to give me two dollars? I'd like to buy a candle to light so I can say a prayer to the Virgin Mother."

I pressed two one-dollar bills into her hand, and she shuffled away.

A week or so later, I returned to the grotto to pray. An afternoon shower dampened the stone steps in places. As I was trying to side-step some puddles, that same woman came up to me again.

"I feel guilty," she began, her head hung low. "That two dollars you gave me to buy a candle? Well, I used the money to buy a slice of pizza and a soda."

I smiled and touched her on the shoulder. "You must have been hungry, and the money and food were answers to your prayers."

I was trying to remember all my heavenly teachings, and I thought that my response is what Jesus would have wanted me to tell her.

"Thank you, sir!" Her eyes filled with tears.

We stood there together for a few moments, our heads bowed in prayer, and I noticed that my left foot was in one of the puddles. As I moved my foot out of it, the woman pointed down and screamed: "Look down!"

There, imprinted on the stone floor, was the image of a crucifix. It was unmistakable, clear as day. The cross was a Celtic cross, a magnificent image that lasted for a few minutes before evaporating from view. Together, gasping in amazement, we went inside to the interior chapel and fell to our knees in prayer. We both knew we had just witnessed a miracle.

It wasn't long before I was given a second miracle at the very same site. After seeing the cross imprinted on the stone floor, I found ways to go back to the grotto each week to pray. On one particular day, I arrived at dusk. I was waiting for someone to come and lock up the shrine but nobody came, so I continued my devotions. As I finished my prayers, I looked up and saw a golden light in front of me that soon turned into an image of a woman resembling Mother Mary. As I stared, my attention riveted, I could make out a baby in her arms. There were four other men standing with her.

Bathed in golden light, Mother Mary began to talk to me telepathically as Jesus did in Heaven. She told me that the baby was Jesus; the man beside her was her husband, Joseph; and behind him were the three wise men who came to honor Jesus at His birth. Mother Mary then looked up and pointed to the sky. I raised my eyes to the sky and saw a brilliant star appear. This was the Star of Bethlehem, she told me, the same star that appeared the night that Jesus was born. The beautiful star was unlike any I have ever seen before or since. I could clearly make out 18 distinct spokes of brilliant light emanating from its center. It was breathtakingly beautiful, just like Mother Mary herself.

I couldn't believe my eyes!

I was flooded with warmth, and I began to sob. My heart filled up with the same love and peace that I felt when I was in Heaven. We were there together for what seemed like hours.

Then, in an instant, I felt something change inside me, as if something was being released. It was the pain leaving my body! For the first time since I had returned from Heaven, I felt no pain, anywhere.

I sobbed even harder. I was experiencing a miracle. As the vision of Mother Mary faded, I collapsed on a bench, feeling completely filled with Divine Unconditional Love.

CHAPTER
13

RECOVERING

SEVERAL MONTHS AFTER THE miracle at the grotto, I began working on strengthening my body to speed my recovery. I started a workout program and a new food plan. I remembered how light I felt in Heaven; I wanted to feel that way here on Earth.

Although I kept to myself and told no one about what happened to me, I definitely felt different. I was more peaceful, grateful, and aware. I noticed how connected everything was, and I didn't go through a single day without seeing tiny miracles. To this day, my eyes are open to God's divine hand in all things, and I see what I would surely have missed before the accident.

I began to see butterflies flying all around me. I watched the birds in the sky. I noticed the grass and the flowers and their beauty. The trees seemed like my friends. I often stopped to touch them and bond with them, because now I knew that they could feel me and that my connection to them helped us both. All trees share a consciousness, and their purpose is to oxygenate the air we breathe. They provide us with shade, with food, with grace, and with love.

One day I was sitting in a park. A kid started whacking a tree with his baseball bat. With every strike of the bat, I felt the tree's pain. I got up and asked the boy, "Do you know the tree feels pain when you hit it?"

"Really?" he asked, wide-eyed. He put down his bat and hugged the tree.

In the evenings, I made it a habit to stargaze. I never took time for this before. Now I tried not to miss an opportunity to see the phases of the moon and the stars twinkling. I never saw the Star of Bethlehem again, but I know it's up there somewhere, and that gives me great comfort even today.

When it rained, I waited to see if I could catch a glimpse of a rainbow. Rainbows in Heaven are truly spectacular, but any rainbow anywhere is magical. Rainbows connect us to God's handiwork.

On the weekends, I went to the beach. After the ocean experience with Jesus in Heaven, I felt compelled to ground myself in the ocean waters. I loved sitting by the sea, becoming part of its rhythm. I loved the way the hot sun felt on my skin, and I liked watching all the sea life make its way in and out of the water.

I had been changed! I was very different from the man I was prior to the near-death experience. I could see and feel the vibration and energy of everything around me. I knew for certain that there is no death and that I came back with new gifts that were astonishing to this simple man with no college education and no medical training whatsoever.

The first new gift I noticed right away was the deep connection I felt to every living thing. I felt connected to people, to animals, to plants, the ocean, and of course, all the flowers and trees. I could feel the Vital Force vibrating all around me. I was a part of it all and connected through all my senses. I could actually sense and feel love pulsating within all living things. In my mind, I could see how everything is all connected, even if our eyes see things around us as separate, discrete objects. That separation is an illusion; we are all connected to each other and to everything in nature and on the planet. I remembered that connection was the first revelation that Jesus taught me because it is the foundation for all other knowledge.

As I interacted with people, I discovered that I could see within a person in ways that were impossible before the accident. Jesus had told me I was becoming more and this certainly was "more." It was almost like I had X-ray vision or something.

My near-death experience had altered and widened my perceptions to such a degree that I was able to see the state of a person's health. I could "tune in," particularly to areas of health or mental and emotional anguish and grief. I couldn't read minds, but I could feel beyond a person's words. It was like I could access a blueprint of a person's body and know intuitively what the problem areas were. I could sense emotional and physical pain, heartache, inflammation, injury, and disease. I could see if a person was filled with light and love and faith, or if they were lost or suffering and alone in their beliefs.

I was also able to assess a person's capacity for healing based on the vibration of their mind, body, and spirit. Jesus really emphasized how we all have the capacity to self-heal, and I could see blockages in people's energy fields just by looking at them. I could tell a person's capacity to emanate Divine Unconditional Love. I don't have great eyes, but my "inner vision" was certainly 20/20! I "saw" and felt more than ever before.

I also could perceive auras around people. Jesus had described our electromagnetic nature when he taught me the Revelation of Grounding. The reason we can use the Earth to ground ourselves and detoxify our bodies is because we are electromagnetic and so is the Earth. That energy produces an aura that some human beings can perceive. These auras surround us and change color to reflect our state of being at any given moment.

I also discovered that my intuition seemed stronger and enhanced. I felt like I was plugged in to universal truths and knew how things worked much differently than before. As a plumber, I understood how water flowed through pipes, how blockages occurred, and how to increase water pressure and flow. If you think of human health and the role energy plays in our abilities to heal ourselves, it's really not that different. The higher our vibration, the more energy can flow through our bodies comfortably without blockage. This makes it easier for the body to detoxify and process out the elements that hurt our health.

The next and most important feeling within myself was a deep sense of gratitude. Because I was more connected than ever before, I noticed all the little miracles around me that I took for granted or didn't stop to notice before my accident. The beauty of nature, the butterflies, the blue skies, the rainbows, the wonderful smell of freshly cut grass, the sounds of the ocean, the birds . . . I saw and felt it all and it all felt like a miracle. How could all of this have slipped by me before? It was almost as if I had been sleepwalking and not aware of the world and its magnificence. I had always been pretty upbeat and social but I think I was missing some of the awe and wonder that surrounded me every single day. Now, I saw it all. I was awake and truly alive.

I thought often about how Jesus told me He was imprinting His teachings onto my brain so that I could become more. I still wasn't sure what "more" meant, but I could see that my senses had been heightened and my perceptions had been widened.

Mother Mary alleviated my physical pain, but my body was still healing from the broken bones and fractures I had sustained. Yet after several months, I no longer felt unsteady and unsure about being back here. I had returned feeling sorry for myself and way too immersed in my own situation. Now, as the teachings filled me again, I couldn't seem to focus on just myself. Jesus's training had profoundly and fundamentally changed how I looked at everything and everyone.

It was like being reborn.

The Gift of Understanding

My spirits stayed high, but my physical recovery was slow. I decided that if I could practice stillness, I could learn more about why I came back and why I was chosen to have the experience.

And then there was another sign.

I was sitting at my desk at home in prayer and meditation. All of a sudden, I felt this amazing force, some incredible energy coming toward me. The energy felt familiar, like the energy I felt in Heaven and at the grotto—a very high vibration of Divine Unconditional Love. I couldn't see the energy, but I could feel it as something very powerful but also very warm and loving, just like in Heaven.

Minutes later, I saw a large, bright ball of blue light come through the wall and streak through my apartment from one end to the other. The power of this blue ball of light made the lights in my apartment and the entire neighborhood go dark. All I could see was this amazing light. After a few minutes, the blue energy ball disappeared. The lights in my apartment and the neighborhood came back on. After witnessing this energy appear and disappear, I felt stronger and somehow revitalized. I felt even more connected to everything and more comfortable in my body.

Hidden in that ball was the gift of understanding. It was in this unforgettable moment that I received divine guidance and the answer that I had been seeking since I returned from Heaven. The reason I came back was so that I could someday share the revelations about how to access divine healing and help people better understand the nature of health and healing.

There was a reason—a plan—for why I was hit by a car, delivered to Heaven, and patiently taught precious revelations by Jesus. I was given the ability to see the new purpose for my life. I was meant to be able to understand the complexities of energy, learn how to self-heal, and help people understand that death isn't something to fear.

To honor what I was learning, I settled into as much of a routine as possible. I prayed and meditated every day. I expressed gratitude. I continued to eat cleanly, meaning no processed foods or artificial ingredients. I monitored my thoughts for negativity, which I knew would produce only bad outcomes. Through faithfulness, positivity, and self-love, I became the architect of my own reality.

With all these new ideas and insights flowing into me, my spirit was soaring, but there was a negative side. I began to realize that my relationships prior to the accident had fallen by the wayside, most certainly because I was a changed man, unrecognizable to those who knew me before. Loneliness and isolation set in and began to grow.

I suspect they grew because I kept to myself. I didn't share my experience with anyone. I thought it would sound too crazy, too over the top. I couldn't imagine going up to someone new and saying, "Oh, yeah, I died and came back, and by the way, I met Jesus and God, and they taught me about the purpose of life and how to create a divinely inspired life." Hearing that, who wouldn't think I was crazy, self-righteous, or self-important? Down deep, I was just afraid of being ridiculed. Despite my trip to Heaven, I was still imperfectly human.

As time went on, though, I realized I was continuing to struggle with my old issues of self-worth, self-love, and balance. Maybe my reluctance to share my story also stemmed from the fact that I didn't always honor my miracle. My life had many unhealed aspects, and there were stumbling blocks ahead.

CHAPTER
14

THE FALL

IN THE EIGHTH YEAR following the accident and my NDE, I hit a mental and emotional wall. Old habits crept in. My health became less of a priority. I didn't go to the beach like I used to, nor did I make time to grocery shop, so I ate out a lot and made bad food choices. I ate too much sugar and gobbled up whatever was available.

I didn't exercise enough, either. My only activity was shifting from one seated position to another. At night, I slouched in a chair, where I fell asleep watching TV until something or some dream startled me awake. Then I stumbled upstairs into my empty bed. Not a lot of movement or self-care in that routine! Those days of sitting and praying and meditating at the grotto seemed very distant. I became seriously imbalanced. I put on more than a hundred pounds.

Jesus had placed into my brain precious knowledge about energy, frequency, vibration, human anatomy, physiology, and toxic threats, as well as information to elevate my well-being on so many levels. But this divine knowledge didn't include an owner's manual. There were no directions for using the information I was given.

My increased awareness and intuition were wonderful gifts—beyond wonderful, really—and I so cherished being able to feel the connections between people. However, I just couldn't seem to make the personal connections myself, the way I used to. I was lonely and purposely keeping myself isolated. I became reclusive.

I wanted to integrate the revelations into my new life, but I didn't believe in myself the way God and His Son believed in me. Despite all the heavenly assurances, in my human heart and mind, I felt that I wasn't worthy of what had happened to me. I wondered if other NDErs felt the same way. I never joined any NDE groups or got counseling, because I just wanted to keep the experience to myself.

But then, one more time, God showed me how much He loves me. He placed my future wife, Michelle, directly in my path.

Several months into my backslide, my good friend Nancy sensed my loneliness and my downward spiral. She introduced me to Michelle, thinking that we would have much in common. Was she ever on the mark! It was a life-changing introduction, and Michelle and I are both forever grateful to our mutual friend.

When I met Michelle, I felt the strongest connection that I ever felt with anyone in my life—so comfortable, in fact, that, soon after meeting her, I was able to tell her about my experience. She didn't freak out or think I was crazy. Conversely, she confided that she was born with special gifts of her own that she didn't talk about, either, unless she developed trust in a person.

Michelle, I learned, is very spiritual and close to God. She is an intuitive and has been talking to God ever since she can remember. She says that there is no time that she is aware of that God hasn't been a part of her life. She grew up in a very religious Orthodox Jewish family, and her mother kept a kosher house. Michelle began having conversations with Jesus when she was a little girl. Jesus and God became her lifeline. God is her center, her essence. As she explains it, she doesn't really know where God stops and she begins. It is all one to her. They are one.

She had had her own hardships, including a rough, abusive childhood; a difficult protracted illness; and her own brush with death. She understood my life. Michelle believes that a successful life is dedicated to two things: faith and love. Nothing else really matters. From faith and love, everything else flows. It is because of who she is and how she lives that Michelle understood me so completely.

We both lived in Florida but 200 miles apart. We saw each other as much as possible, but on a day-to-day basis I was still alone and missing her. She had a certain peace within her that inspired me whenever we were together. At those times, I ate better and took better care of myself. She made me laugh, and I sure needed some laughter in my life.

When Michelle was not around, I reverted to eating poorly. I didn't do anything about my weight. I couldn't seem to make a lasting commitment to get back on a healthy track on my own.

Then, one day, it suddenly happened. I was once again saved by the Divine Hand.

I was helping a neighbor with a home-improvement project when I started to feel really warm and began sweating profusely. I excused myself and headed for the bathroom. An unfamiliar feeling washed over me, and something told me that what was happening was very serious. I splashed water on my face, but I still felt very strange.

All of a sudden, I fell to the bathroom floor. I was having real trouble breathing and could barely catch my breath. I forced myself to stand up and struggled to find my neighbor. I hobbled over to where he was standing but collapsed again in front of him. Fortunately for me, he dialed 911.

Within what seemed like minutes, I could see and feel paramedics working on me as I lay on the floor. My heart was racing madly and felt like it would break out of my chest. The paramedics determined that my heart was in what they call "V-tach," short for *ventricular tachycardia*, an abnormally high heart rate that can deteriorate into life-threatening ventricular fibrillation at any moment. They shocked me with paddles right there on the floor, trying to get my heart back into a normal rhythm. Then they placed me on a stretcher, and I was carted away to the hospital by ambulance.

I was back in a hospital, hooked up to monitors, once again in intensive care. I had wires and cords and IVs and the all-too-familiar hospital wristband. The doctors informed me that I was in pretty bad shape. I had hypertension (high blood pressure), dilated cardiomyopathy (a stretched, enlarged, and weakened heart muscle), and congestive heart failure. I was close to dying—again.

With all my extra weight, there was enormous pressure on my imperfect heart. One of the doctors suggested stomach-stapling surgery so that I could get on a weight-loss fast track in hopes of quickly relieving pressure on my heart. But I rejected that idea because I realized it was a quick fix and wouldn't alleviate my underlying issues.

In addition, my dilated heart muscle contributed to a cardiac arrhythmia called atrial fibrillation, so my heart wasn't pumping blood efficiently. Blood would pool in the chambers of my heart, creating the potential for stroke. My heart's ejection fraction—that is, the percentage of blood pumped out with each contraction— was only 15 percent. Normal is about 50 to 55 percent. A pacemaker and medications helped regulate my erratic heartbeats. I was prescribed additional drugs to help prevent future episodes of congestive heart failure.

My doctor wanted to place me on the heart-transplant waiting list. His message was loud and clear: The heart does not heal and does not regenerate itself. At best, the doctors could keep it from getting worse.

When I heard that, I knew that I'd rather die than have my heart replaced with someone else's; I knew intuitively that I wasn't done with this one. This heart, however damaged, needed to overcome a lack of self-love and a lingering feeling of unworthiness that, forgive the pun, was at the heart of the matter.

All the gloom and doom about my quality of life and the options presented made my imperfect, unhealed heart sink further. Cardiologist after cardiologist gave me the same bad news: My heart condition could not improve.

But here's what I knew: I had survived someone pulling the trigger of a gun multiple times into the back of my head. I had survived being run over. When it was declared that I would never walk again, I defied the odds and did indeed walk again. Scary odds were just that—odds—and odds could be overcome. I had done it before. I could do it again.

I was determined to prove the medical experts wrong. Jesus had taught me so much about healing. Even though I had let my own healing slip away, I believed in my heart that my own heart could heal and get better and stronger. I knew miracles were real. My time in Heaven had been a miracle.

I consciously made the decision to save myself right then and there. This time I wanted to live. I wasn't ready to go home, as beautiful as Heaven is.

I wanted the joy of watching people get second chances, just like I had. I wanted to see if my relationship with Michelle could blossom into something more. I wanted more time, and I was ready to fight for it.

But it would be a tough fight.

Healing Love

For me, the most healing factor was the unconditional love offered to me by Michelle. She agreed to put her life aside to be with me.

Out of pure, selfless love, Michelle took a leave of absence from her job and stayed by my bedside day after day, night after night. She asked my nurses to roll in a sleeping recliner so she could stay with me all night. While I was in intensive care, she slept in the hallway because of the strictly enforced visiting hours. After I was finally transferred to a regular room, she slept next to me, often holding my hand. Michelle would roam the hallways trying to find the largest hospital gowns that would cover my extra-wide girth. She soothed me, prayed with me, and made me laugh even when the doctors were not hopeful.

You know from your own life when you are in the presence of someone who brings out the best in you and loves you dearly. You are filled with joy, happiness, and pure love. Jesus talked about the power of relationships in Heaven as one of the strongest vehicles for spiritual growth. It is such a precious gift when you connect with someone who really "gets" you. That's how I felt with Michelle. I had fallen deeply in love with her, and I knew I wanted to marry her. But I needed to get myself truly back on track and recommit to my life and those revelations before I could commit to her.

There was another person who came into my life at this difficult time: Susan, a friend I came to regard like a sister. I had met Susan at a health-food store that was hosting a mini seminar on the benefits of nutritional supplements. She was very knowledgeable about health and alternative medicine. We quickly felt a strong mutual connection.

After I became ill, Susan rushed to my help as well. She and her daughters, whom I think of as my nieces (they call me Uncle Tommy), stayed with me throughout my ordeal. So there I found myself with two wonderful women who loved one another and loved me, and they worked heartfully together to help me overcome my health issues.

After a long hospitalization, I was finally released in hopes that I could remain in a stable condition. I was grateful to be out on my own again and determined to conquer my demons.

As the weeks went by, my body started to stabilize. I had a laundry list of medicines. I needed a portable oxygen tank with me when I moved around. But I was moving around, even if only slowly at first and with help.

What happened next illustrates beautifully the Revelation of Connection.

Susan knew of a doctor, a cardiologist near her home in Connecticut, who was and still is quite well-known. She had heard him speak on the radio and seen him on television and was very impressed by him. The doctor's name: Stephen Sinatra. One day, Susan brought me a copy of a book he had written, entitled *Metabolic Cardiology*. Because I had so much time on my hands, I read it cover to cover. I was mesmerized.

In that book, Dr. Sinatra talks about healing the heart. He includes many case studies of patients who'd followed his protocol and significantly improved their heart function. This was a very different message than what I had been hearing from my own doctors. They didn't believe that the heart could regenerate. The best they could do was to medicate me to keep my condition from getting worse. Dr. Sinatra's message was revolutionary by comparison. He was saying exactly what I believed: that the heart could heal.

And more than that, he laid out a specific program to follow to accomplish just that—heart healing! I was surprised by its simplicity: a combination of nutritional supplements that he referred to as the Awesome Foursome. They were CoQ10, magnesium, carnitine, and d-ribose.

Dr. Sinatra, I learned, had written other books about heart health. I bought and read them as well, and then I subscribed to his monthly newsletter. His words gave me hope! I began to follow his protocol precisely.

With a new mind-set toward healing myself, I tapped into an old friend of mine, Joe Bucci, a former Mr. World who took excellent care of himself. Joe connected me to a fitness-and-nutrition expert who had trained many famous actors for their action-movie roles. This expert tested my blood and prescribed a diet unique to my blood type and food preferences. I began to follow it religiously, eating nothing other than what was on the program.

Good-bye, pizza! Hello, broccoli!

Finally, I felt as though I was putting into practice the lessons that Jesus had shared with me about caring for my physical body. I was able to commit these radical changes to my lifestyle and diet because at last I felt that I was on the path I was meant to take.

Days turned into weeks; weeks turned into months. The going was tough, but I was determined to overcome the hurdles. My life revolved around doctors' appointments, medicines, rest, and diet. The weight was beginning to come off, and I was back to eating better—in fact, better than ever—and sleeping many hours. I think God was healing me as I slept, because I could feel myself changing, growing stronger, and becoming more positive.

Michelle had given up her job and her apartment and moved in with me to help me get well. I needed a lot of help. I wasn't very mobile, and I couldn't drive yet. Susan stayed very close to the situation, offering guidance and the latest research and information on heart disease. She championed Dr. Sinatra's approach, and I continued to follow his program.

Everything was working. I lost 140 pounds in nine months!

I still had residual health issues, but I was definitely healing, and I wanted to make Michelle my wife. So, 10 years after my accident, we were quietly married and officially began our life together. We both knew I still had a long road ahead of me, but we were going to approach everything as a team.

One morning I was watching TV, flipping through the channels, and I stumbled onto a cable show on health hosted by former family-practice physician Richard Becker and his wife, Cindy. The show, *Your Health with Dr. Richard and Cindy Becker*, was filled with fascinating information and expertise, a blending of traditional and alternative approaches to fighting disease and regaining wellness. I began to watch regularly for the down-to-earth advice and interviews the show offered. I was surprised one day to tune in and find out that Dr. Sinatra was a guest on the show. Michelle and I were both excited to finally see and hear the doctor whose recommendations I had been following so closely for nearly a year.

Dr. Sinatra's comments resonated totally with me, and one thing he said in particular stands out in my mind as a defining moment in my understanding of what health and healing and the doctor-patient relationship are all about. In response to a question from the Beckers, he said that he considered himself as more of a healer than a doctor, and to be a healer required more than just looking at a person's physiology. To heal, he said, you needed to see the "whole picture."

Until that moment, no doctor I had ever encountered talked that way. The doctors I had met spoke in statistics. There were no gray areas, just black-and-white. I was more than impressed. I was moved.

So was Michelle. Quietly but with great certainty, she said, "Tommy, this is your doctor. This man has been selected by God to help you heal yourself, and more than that, you will become great friends with him. You will help each other. We know him. He is part of our family. We have known him for a very long time."

I looked at her in amazement. Michelle is not given to drama or grandiose statements. Over the years, I've learned to trust her intuition. She is somehow plugged into truths that are powerful and meaningful. So when she spoke with such clarity, I listened and thought about what she was saying. I knew I felt something inside when I heard Dr. Sinatra speak about healing the heart. Maybe it was respect or maybe the excitement of the resonance between him, someone with all those important degrees after his name, and me, with nothing behind my name. Both Michelle and I resonated personally with Dr. Sinatra's reference to himself as a healer. There was definitely a connection. It wasn't just my wife feeling it; I could feel it, too.

I continued following his program and my diet plan. I had lost the weight I needed to take off, but I was still a healing work in progress. There were missing pieces, some fine-tuning that needed to occur before I'd allow myself to get back into the full swing of things.

As I worked on forming better habits and following up self-love practices, Michelle watched over me like a fierce protectress.

It was about a year later, in 2010, when we learned that Dr. Sinatra would be speaking at a conference in Saint Petersburg, Florida. At that time, attending a medical conference seemed daunting to me. I was still not 100 percent by any means. Although I was off the oxygen tank and moving a lot better, I was still on medication and tired easily. Michelle, however, felt that something important would happen if we went. I knew that if I let fear in, fear would take over. So, reluctantly, I agreed to go.

There were fascinating topics to choose from, as well as a spacious exhibit hall where vendors displayed their health-care products and shared the latest technology in health and healing. I signed up for a few lectures, including Dr. Sinatra's.

His topic was "Earthing" and the importance of connecting ourselves to the Earth regularly to better maximize our health and sleep, as well as reduce our accumulated burden of pain, inflammation, and toxicity.

Sound familiar?

I was amazed to hear this traditionally trained cardiologist cite science and empirical data that confirmed the specifics I had learned in Heaven! Jesus had talked extensively about the need to ground ourselves to the Earth in order to clear out toxins and radiation. And here was Dr. Sinatra telling the audience the very same thing!

After the lecture concluded, I went up to our room to take a break. Michelle was waiting for me, eager to hear about my morning.

"I find it amazing," I told her, "that I was able to follow everything that the lecturers were saying, even though I never went to college or opened a medical book."

It wasn't ego. I wasn't bragging. I was simply expressing my gratitude regarding the magnitude of the gift I had received in Heaven.

Michelle just smiled and said, "Tommy, God put everything you needed to know inside of you before you came back from Heaven.

That is the miracle. You were meant to be able to understand the complexities of energy, how to self-heal, and to help people understand that death isn't something to fear. Heaven is our real home. You shouldn't feel bad about not going to college. You went to Divine University—the Heavenly Institute. You had the best teacher ever: Jesus. Isn't that better?"

We ran into Dr. Sinatra after his presentation as he was resting his hip, and began to talk. Michelle told me afterward that she "just knew" our meeting was important and left me to plant the seeds of a friendship she believed was divinely inspired.

I connected with Dr. Sinatra and his wife, Jan, over dinner when they passed through our hometown not long after the conference. Unfortunately, Michelle couldn't join me, so I went off solo to share with them the story of how the doctor's protocol had truly saved my life for the second time.

I could see that the Sinatras are a dynamic couple, functioning as a team in much the same way that Michelle and I operate together. They love each other very much and are devoted to family and work, and their life revolves around service to others. They are dedicated to teaching people how to attain good health. It didn't take long for me to realize that these two extraordinary people have been walking the same path that Jesus laid out for me in Heaven.

Steve and Jan had already incorporated the precious lessons I learned into their lives and work. Spending time with them, I felt a great sense of closeness. We were kindred souls. Despite our obvious differences in education and training, I sensed we were establishing a rewarding, lifelong friendship.

Dr. Sinatra and I had many extraordinary conversations about my experience in Heaven and what I learned about health from Jesus. With every word I spoke, he was astonished, and vice versa. Our shared attitudes about connection, faithfulness, grounding, Vital Force, and the other revelations were more than mere coincidences—they were miraculous in the way they matched exactly what he practiced on

Earth. We both believed—and knew for sure—that by applying these revelations in a practical way, many people could prevent, even heal, very serious diseases.

We also had many discussions about what happens when someone is ready to "cross over," and these were meaningful, eye-opening conversations. In our society, death has many faces. Unfortunately, our modern, high-tech society has made death something of a taboo, keeping it at a distance as though it were some foreign invader rather than an integral, expected, and normal part of life.

We both agree that death should not be viewed in such an alien, let's-not-talk-about-it, don't-want-to-face-it kind of way. Instead, Dr. Sinatra and I feel that we must transform the final chapter of our life, the conclusion of our time here on Earth, from a frightening experience into a spiritual awakening. For when we each face up to our own mortality, the process of dying can be a truly spiritual and healing experience, for both the dying person and the surrounding loved ones.

As a cardiologist, Dr. Sinatra has been at the bedside of many people in their final moments. He told me, "It always amazes me how peaceful a dying person can look in the presence of loved ones. I have found that when the family is able to unselfishly support what I call the deathing process, all may attain a common bond of spiritual liberation."

Keep in mind that to die means not only losing our bodies, minds, physical possessions, and relationships but also facing our deepest fears, including loss of control and fear of the unknown. In this extremely vulnerable position, the dying person may experience panic and guilt, as well as repressed emotions, including anger and jealousy toward those who will continue to live. Even in a coma or a semicoma, such emotions may surface. The dying person may not want to die or may be regretful about something that happened in the past. It is here where so many of the revelations from my Teacher can come back into play; it is never too late to begin practicing them in earnest. Whatever the emotions—whether sadness, anger, or surrender—it is extremely important to encourage their release when they arise.

Dr. Sinatra told me that because hearing is the last sense to fade away, sound can be very important to the dying person. Soothing music can be of an enormous comfort, as can reading or reciting scripture. It is always best if the music or sounds you select have special meaning for the dying person. Patients and coaches can also recite positive affirmations that are consistent with their belief system. Christians, for example, can say, "Lord Jesus, have mercy on me." Those of the Jewish faith can chant, "Hear O Israel, the Lord our God, the Lord is one." And people of all faiths can say, "Into thy hands I commend my soul."

Dr. Sinatra also revealed to me the common body sensations signaling death's imminent approach. Such symptoms can include:

- Overwhelming fatigue

- A sinking or floating sensation

- Alternative feelings of hot or cold

- A softening of the body

- Heaviness in the body

- A sense of profound peacefulness

- Shallow breathing

- Dizziness

- Disorientation

- Seemingly odd images and visions

- Talking or mumbling in a strange language

- Sudden cessation of breathing followed by gasps for air

Finally, when you believe the moment of death is at hand, while giving your loving touch, you may want to say words like these:

"My dear, I love you very much and I will miss you. Have no fear and let everything happen naturally. Look for a light and think pleasant thoughts." Dr. Sinatra revealed that saying these words frequently over and over again can give comfort to not only the one leaving but to all others at the bedside.

I've always cherished these discussions with Dr. Sinatra and his wife, and I always look forward to our next conversation, whether it is about health, the revelations, Heaven, or what is going on in our lives. I feel uplifted with the Sinatras because our time together gives me a chance to reflect on the revelations and discover new ways to actively live them. Meeting the Sinatras has been another divine gift and further proof that we are all connected.

I remember one evening, as we parted ways, Jan spontaneously lowered her head and placed a kiss directly on my heart. No one before in my life had ever done anything like that. It flooded my heart with the purest healing love.

I consider the friendship I have with Jan and Steve Sinatra one of the happiest blessings since my return to life. The way the four of us (I am including my wife, Michelle) understand death and live life ties directly back to the precious revelations I was given in Heaven. We live our life's purpose in service to God and humanity as much as possible. We ground to the Earth every day. We eat clean diets, we pray, meditate, and give thanks for our blessings. We practice self-love and try to Be Love every day. In this way, we keep our vibrations high and stave off aging and disease.

We enjoy our deep friendship with each other and others and most of all we feel blessed. We have the knowledge that there is no real death and when our time comes, it will be like walking through a door to our real "Home."

All I know is that when I see my Heavenly Father again at the end of my life and He asks me, "Son, what did you do with the gifts that I gave you?" I want to have a good answer. I want to be able to proudly tell my Heavenly Father, "I used everything, all of it, and I did it in Your Name."

CHAPTER
15

LIFE AS THE
NEW TOMMY

YEARS AFTER I CAME back from Heaven, an amazing and unexpected event happened. It helped reaffirm my faith in what happened to me. I took Michelle to my old neighborhood in the Bronx. She said she wanted to see where I used to live, but I think she was more curious about the accident and where I was struck down. Not in a morbid way—I think she wanted to see if she could "feel" anything if she saw the place where it happened. Neither of us was prepared for what happened next.

When we reached my old apartment house, I slowed down and parked the car. Without saying a word, Michelle walked right over to where I had been hit by the car and "died." She just stood over the spot and trembled as big tears rolled down her face.

"I can feel everything, Tommy, like it just happened," she declared as she wiped her tears away with her sleeve. More than 15 years had passed. I had never been back until now. I didn't know what I would feel or what to expect, so I just hadn't visited. Now that I was standing on the very spot where the car had hit me, I didn't feel sad or scared. I just felt happy that I was alive, that this was my past and I have a new life with someone who really loves me.

During our years together, I had never really sat down and told my story in a linear fashion to Michelle—or anyone else, for that matter. I would just describe a little bit here, a little bit there. I had shared the health revelations that I learned in Heaven with Jan and Steve Sinatra, but I had never told the full story in a sequential way until I sat down to write it for this book.

After a few minutes of Michelle energetically "reliving" my accident, she became anxious to move around. She noticed the old corner store and said she was going in to get us some water. I didn't say anything to her. I hadn't been in that store since before the accident. As she went inside, she made small talk with the man at the register. She asked him casually how long he had been there. He replied that he owned the store and had been there for more than 15 years.

On a whim, Michelle asked him if he remembered an accident that occurred across the street. He looked startled for a moment. Then his eyes widened and he seemed excited to tell my wife what he remembered about that night.

The merchant, Carlos, a sweet older man, responded to Michelle: "Yes, I remember that night! I will never forget it. A man, one of my regular customers, was making his way across the street. He was coming to my store when a car with no lights on appeared out of nowhere and was going very fast. The car hit the man and sped away without stopping.

"I saw the man lying on the ground. He wasn't moving at all, so I thought for sure he was dead. I called 911 and as I was waiting for help, I saw something happen that I have never forgotten, and I have told no one about this. They would think I am crazy!"

Michelle listened as my story unfolded.

"I saw the man's spirit rise up from his body. His spirit was white, and I saw it lift up from his body. It was dark because it was late at night, but I know what I saw. The man was very still and his spirit was very white, but I could see through it. His spirit lifted up. Then it was gone! I couldn't see it anymore. That's when I knew the man was dead. He was my customer. He came into my store every night! He was so young!"

My wife couldn't believe what she was hearing. How amazing that not only was the man who witnessed the accident still here, but he remembered seeing my spirit rise up from my body! Excitedly, she told the merchant that the very same customer was her husband and not only wasn't he dead—he was outside! She motioned wildly for me to come inside.

As I entered that store, all of my old memories flooded back in a rush. It was so good to see Carlos again! And he was very happy to see that I was alive!

In truth, I am more alive now than I was before my "death."

I'll bet that if you could get a whole bunch of folks who had experienced a near-death together in the same room, they would tell you that there is a definite difference between life before a near-death experience and life after one.

The NDE changes you. I know that it changed me. Based on what I have read about NDEs, I've learned that it is not unusual for people to come back with new gifts and insights. Some people come back with more intuition, as I did; some, with more artistic or musical ability. Others return as mediums or channels with the ability to communicate with those who have passed over.

I knew the Old Tommy to be a nice guy, a pretty ordinary fellow with a big heart. He would give you the shirt off his back. If you needed a few bucks or a ride somewhere or help with a project, he was your man. Old Tommy was a good pal and a decent plumber—an average guy trying to do his best every day.

As New Tommy, I know that I have been changed for the better. I can't talk to dead people or fly or levitate or anything spectacular like that, but I know there is more to me than before. As I mentioned earlier, I'm more in tune with people. I was friendly before, but now I savor every opportunity to form a connection. I take the time to say "good morning" and "God bless you" and "thank you" more often.

I know that I have been forever changed. Instead of being impatient, blind, or bothered by things in life, I embrace everything positively. No longer do I think of just myself. I am everyone and everyone is me. I can still hear Jesus in my head, echoing all of our lessons, constantly reminding me that we are all truly connected.

What a heart-touching honor and privilege it is to have had Jesus give me the tiniest glimpse into God's intention for our lives and our development. Based on my experience, I know that God has a plan for me and for everyone else. We just have to seek stillness and try to hear what God is saying to us about what He would like us to do. God has a hand in everything. Our challenge is to realize God is in control, listen to Him, and be obedient to what He is asking of us.

I have had a lot of time to reflect on what Jesus revealed to me, and I'm thankful to have learned the eight revelations. I see that they are powerful truths that increase our vibration and thus promote health and healing. But I also realize that they build on each other, and, like everything else in the universe, connect with each other. They give us the meaning and context we need for mind, body, and spiritual health and healing.

The healing we need begins with connection. We're divinely programmed to seek relationships, and the quality of those relationships affects our health. But fear and lack of faith can keep us from reaching out. We need faith, especially when we get to the difficult parts of our lives, because it cancels out fear, gives our life a deeper meaning, and expands and deepens our connections. Faith in ourselves and in God helps us live out every one of the revelations and directs the course we take in life.

There's a Vital Force pulsating through us, governing all interactions and the essence of life. Our choices, from what we eat to how we think to what we believe, support our Vital Force and lead to vibrant health and energy. Even the very Earth on which we live has a Vital Force—an electromagnetic energy that, when absorbed in the body through grounding, promotes better health in many different ways. Grounding helps rid the body of physical toxins, as does choosing high-vibration foods that protect the temple that is the body.

I've learned that many illnesses can be traced back to things like heavy metals, fungi, bacteria, viruses, parasites, radiation, immunizations, chemicals, and flukes (microscopic parasites living in food and water). All these factors have their own specific frequency and vibration. We get sick as a result of our personal vibration becoming depleted. That can happen if we disrespect our bodies—our temples—by eating poorly, taking drugs, drinking too much alcohol, becoming exhausted, or getting into a negative mental or emotional state that keeps us out of touch with our divine connections.

Some of us have stronger immune systems than others. Why is this so? There are many factors that explain the differences in immune system strength. It could be genetics, lifestyle choices, or negative mental thinking. When a person's vibration isn't high enough to stave off one of these conditions, a virus, bacteria, or a parasite opportunistically enters the physical system and runs amok. It gravitates to the weakest part of the body and then works to replicate itself in order to survive. If your vibration is higher than that of any opportunistic offender, then the invader cannot survive and will perish without causing damage to your body. A high vibration creates and sustains a healthy immune system.

Just as there are physical toxins, there are mental ones, too. They can be cleared by positivity in thought. Positivity also brings to us what we seek and what we think optimistically about—the good in life. Through positivity, we can begin to develop greater self-love. Self-love is the first step on the path to loving relationships, affection, and self-care and the ability to give and receive unconditional love. Our lives ultimately become an expression of that unconditional love.

Because God treats me so tenderly, I need to treat myself the same way. I must be gentle toward the places in myself that have been wounded. I can release the lie I've often told myself—that I have to be perfect to be loved. I can accept the gift of unconditional love that God gives freely to me, with no strings attached. And I can love others in the same way.

As I learned in Heaven, we are what we think, what we believe, and what we choose. We honor or dishonor our divine and human connections with every decision we make personally and collectively. We would have such a beautiful world if we could all be on Earth as it is in Heaven.

When we listen to our hearts, we can discover our true reason and mission for being on this planet and how to use our gifts and talents to express that true mission with authenticity and freedom. It comforts me to know that our lives are meant to be purposeful.

This key to health and life is exactly what Jesus explained to me: keeping your vibration as high as possible. And we can also do that by applying the eight revelations.

As I journeyed through Heaven and heard the eight revelations, all I knew was that I loved being there. I was humbled and grateful to know that I have a guardian angel, a spiritual helper looking after me who is involved in my life and cares about my well-being. I loved being with Jesus, who was my Teacher and guide. I felt love from him toward me, and I was filled with love for him. It was more love than I've ever felt for anyone in my whole life, including myself.

I know you might be wondering about the Jesus I met. What if you are a follower of a different faith? Since I've been back from

Heaven, I've wondered the same thing. What about others who go to Heaven? Whom do they meet?

Even though it has been years since my accident, I have often thought of Jesus telling me that there is no wrong way to love God, and that there are a thousand paths to His door. After all, we are all children of God, and we all have that part of God that lives within us—that Divine Spark.

I grew up as a Catholic so I suppose it was natural for me to meet Jesus in Heaven. Did God choose Jesus to be my guide and teacher because Jesus is an important part of my faith? I remember Jesus saying:

> *Faith should not separate people, but instead should bind them together to God. Belief systems, however diverse they may seem, are all rooted in God's love. All faiths should be respected and honored.*

His answer now makes sense to me. Perhaps people of different faiths who experience near-death might meet a different Teacher who aligns with their belief systems. They might meet Mother Mary, angels, Moses, Abraham, Buddha, Muhammad, Krishna, or other messengers of God's choosing. This is an extraordinary insight.

With all of the insights I received, I have remained humbled, and I know I have to honor my experience forever. Before this accident and the near-death experience, I was a pretty typical guy, and that included going to Mass regularly. But I probably wasn't as committed as I could have been. Like most people, I was busy working and running a business and just went about my life. Those things edged out a lot of my responsibilities to my physical, emotional, and spiritual selves.

Today, as New Tommy, I appreciate life so much more. It is fleeting and fragile, with both good things and bad, but it is a great gift to be treasured. And we should live it with passion and purpose. But I also know that there is life after this life. And I have seen it.

What I do know is that my life would have taken a distinctly different course had the accident never happened and had I never gone to Heaven. Almost dying helped me learn to really live.

I now realize that the revelations were just the beginning—the foundation on which to build my new life. I remember that Jesus taught me that God selects each of us to receive gifts that we can share with each other. He directs us to use these gifts as we see fit with the hope that we will use these precious gifts to honor Him and to be of service to humanity in some capacity.

Learning through Meditation

Today I stay connected to God and all that is divine by creating still-ness in my life. In daily prayer and meditation, I feel God's presence more clearly. My thoughts connect to heavenly matters and divine directives. I become filled with a knowing that creating stillness, where one creates time with God, is the best way to stay aligned with one's divine purpose and potential.

Each time I meditate, I learn more and I see more. I have been shown that God's Divine Unconditional Love creates healing. I have also been shown that not everyone can be healed. Sometimes it's God's plan for an individual to go through the experience of illness. Perhaps it is because that person will learn a valuable lesson through self-evaluation or awareness that might not take place without the illness. Or maybe the disease will give others who touch the life of the sick person the opportunity to become more compassionate and loving. In some cases, it is adversity that strengthens character, rela-tionships, and personal identity.

I don't know why some people recover from life-threatening situ-ations while others don't. Some of us, it seems, must face difficulties such as illness, pain, or loss during the course of our lives. But I know this: God loves each of us and never abandons us at any moment. We may not always understand the reason for what we are experiencing, but we must trust that all we experience is for our highest and greatest good.

I've learned through meditation that understanding illness is only one aspect of getting healthy and well. Treating your life as the precious gift it is and valuing each day that you are given to honor yourself and God is our true divine purpose. This is why we are here: to learn, to grow, and to love.

You and I are like artists with blank canvases that represent our lives. The paints you use to express yourself fully are your unique gifts and talents that you discover throughout your lifetime. The goal is to live through the heart so that you can honor the divinity within. I know from my time in Heaven that God's love for each of us knows no limits. It is endless, everlasting love. No matter what we face in life, whether it is illness, hardship, fear, sadness, or loss, He is there for each of us.

Sharing My Experience

It took me a long time to get here, but today I share my near-death experience openly. Before, I was too afraid of being judged. That fear gave way to shame that I wasn't brave enough to share my story so people could benefit from what I'd learned in Heaven. My heart wanted to share, but my mind always talked me out of it.

Because I wasn't true to my heart, my heart failed. I wasn't being true to myself. I let my stupid ego and fear get in my way, and I sabotaged everything and fell into self-destructive behavior.

It took me a while to understand that all God really wanted me to do was to love myself as He loves me and as He loves us all. He had shown me His love so many times, yet it was a lesson that took me a long time to truly master. I was so busy either trying to prove myself worthy of these gifts or hiding my experience that

I'd forgotten about the need to balance the energy properly. I let myself go and followed self-doubt all the way to a health crisis, and only then was I able to accept the gifts and responsibilities that I had been given. Just like those scary sharks I experienced in Heaven wouldn't have been necessary if I hadn't been so afraid, I wouldn't have needed a health crisis to give me the right perspective had I only had the healthier self-esteem and self-worth that God wants us all to have.

In thinking about the trajectory of my life, I realized something else, something once again larger than myself. I realized that this is a common stumbling block for many people. The need for approval, to be loved, and to be worthy of love causes many of us to stumble and fall. Jesus talked about this in Heaven, but somewhere along the line, I reverted to my old patterns. He knew this would happen to me if I used my free will to make poor choices. When you do not have a solid foundation of self-love, you seek love from others. No matter how many miracles you experience, you still require approval and acknowledgment from outside sources to assuage your own deep insecurities.

Living this way makes imbalance inevitable.

The good news is that each day brings new hope: new opportunities to regroup, to rethink how you are living, to reconsider what you are choosing, and to change any aspect of your life that is not working. The key is figuring out what needs to be embraced and what needs to be eliminated, and then committing to make it happen.

This is not where God steps in. He is already there! This is where you come in to reclaim, reorganize, rethink, reprioritize, and go forward in a new way.

If I could do it, you can do it, too!

One of the coolest things about being alive is that we can change. We can redefine our destinies and shape our own futures with our choices.

We Don't Really Die

The gifts and intuition that God granted me have grown over time. I've slowly learned what is truly important in life. I've discovered how to embrace my own humanity. I know how to face my fears and to forgive myself when I fail. Most important, I have learned to love myself and see my value in God's universe.

I'm so grateful for my life and what happened to me and for what I've learned and what I continue to learn. Of it all, the most important truth is this:

We don't really die.

There is no death, no true end. In many ways, death is a new beginning. God and Jesus graced me with a glimpse of Heaven. If I could use my near-death experience in the most valuable way for others, it would be to help alleviate people's fear of death. Heaven is home. Just know that when your time comes, you'll be infinitely happy there. Believe me, I would have loved to stay in Heaven if I could, but God had other plans for this simple man who never thought much about the afterlife until he died and came back with the truth.

Today I'm a study in gratitude and truly a blessed man. I love my life, and I believe that coming so close to death multiple times gives me a unique perspective of appreciation for just how fragile and precious life is. I have no fear of death. I imagine that many people who have had near-death experiences and have glimpsed the other side feel the same way. There is nothing to fear. We don't end. We just move into a different state of being. Heaven is paradise. Once you have seen it and been there, you carry that image and those feelings deep inside of you. They don't leave you.

But while we are here in our respective bodies, inhabiting this beautiful planet we call Earth, we need to be mindful that we are just renters. We own nothing material. It all belongs to God—your house, car, clothes, jewels, and art. All of the things you may have painstakingly collected over the course of your life will no doubt be owned or enjoyed by someone else down the road. Maybe it will be your children or your children's children—or maybe it will all be scattered to the four winds.

The land, the seas, the sky, and the stars are here for us to enjoy and treasure during our time on Earth. Our bodies were created to be temporary vessels for our souls, and we must treat them with as much love and respect as God created them to receive. In truth, though, all of that belongs to God as well. There is no point in getting too attached to or upset over "stuff."

In Heaven, I was infused with a universal perspective. Probably all people who go and come back receive this infusion and change accordingly. We likely don't think of time and space in the same way. We realize that there is no separation, that any idea of separation between human beings is an illusion that we've made up. We are all the same! We come from the same source. We are all destined to live, to become what we can become, and then to die and go to the place where our spirits take us.

I don't think like this every day, but these ideas and principles are stored permanently in my heart. They govern my actions and my life choices.

I was Old Tommy before my NDE, and he was a pretty good guy. But I am New Tommy now, and I like him—and my life—a whole lot more!

As New Tommy, I live my life with more awareness and appreciation. Jesus taught me that every day you breathe is a day that you can change. Every day is a chance for rebirth. I love that idea, and I embrace it even when life gets challenging or disappointing.

When the sun rises, it is a new day for us all.

Let me leave you with my divine dream. Read it often, to yourself or aloud, as its words possess a very high vibration that can bring peace, calm, and healing into your life.

The Divine Dream

It took me a long time to remember an important teaching that I was given right before I was sent back through the tunnel of light and into my physical body. Maybe it's the most important teaching of all.

My Teacher taught me that when God created us, He gave each of us something—some quality or gift that makes each of us special and unique, just like a snowflake. He gave no one everything. No individual, no being He has ever made has everything in life. God's divine plan is for each of us to discover and express our special gifts.

He also created us as one universal family. The purpose of our lives is to connect with each other and through the love we create; to become one with each other and with Him.

If He bestowed everything into one being, then that person would need no one else. There would be no need to create the relationships and friendships that are the richest sources of personal and spiritual growth. Instead, in His wisdom, God created each of us with our own special gifts so that we could use our lives to discover and share these blessings with each other and the world.

I often dream of all of humanity sitting at one never-ending table in Heaven. Imagine it with me: We are all there, sharing our lives, our stories, and our gifts with each other. There are no place cards at this table; we are one. There are no separations at this table; there are no leaders. We are not designated or divided by gender, race, religion, age, education, or financial status.

We do not represent any particular state or nation, country, or continent. We are only His children, and we speak only one language, the language of Divine Unconditional Love.

At this heavenly table, we are all equal in God's eyes and in our own. We are laughing and smiling together, simply enjoying the feast that God has set out before us. We are sharing our food, our lives, our words, and our love with each other.

This image never leaves me. I keep it in the back of my mind always as a reminder of my miraculous journey.

Perhaps, as his last gift to me, my Teacher imprinted this aspect of God's divine plan into my mind so that I would remember why I was given another chance at life. I think I came back from Heaven just so that I could share it all with you, and you would have the chance to dream it, too.

After all, we are all connected!

Blessings,
Tommy Rosa

AFTERWORD

Heaven and Earth Truths

By Dr. Stephen Sinatra

IF YOU SEE YOURSELF in the light of the truths that Tommy and I have shared from our experiences, you'll know that you are much more than you think you are. There is a higher spiritual awareness within you and available to you. When you tap into this awareness, you will experience more health, peace, hope, and joy. And you can heal yourself through choice and effort.

In the final analysis, know that, while someday our hearts may stop beating, our spirits live on and go to Heaven, where God and the angels reside and our hearts beat once more—in a new place and a better place.

Strengthen your connections. Replace fearful, negative thinking with conscious optimism. Affirm your own self-worth. Love yourself and others unconditionally. Nourish your body and spirit. Find a spiritual endeavor that gives you inner peace, whether it's meditation or prayer, attending worship services, reading spiritual books, doing yoga, or connecting with nature. Live with purpose, because you have much to give.

Through Tommy's experience, this book has shared the good news that your life can be filled with all the things you want, your vibration can be consistently raised, and you have everything you need to live a healthy, fulfilled life. These truths have been taught to us through the teachings of Jesus, Moses, Buddha, and other ascended masters. They focused on inspiring people to rise to a higher level of spiritual awareness. They encouraged those who felt unworthy to see themselves differently and those with heavy burdens to stand tall and walk confidently. They all embodied faith. They assured people that they had all they needed to survive the tough times and emerge from difficulty even stronger than before. As St. Paul so eloquently revealed in his communications, "When I am strong, I am weak and when I am weak, I am strong."

Ways to Increase Your Vibration

By Dr. Stephen Sinatra

I HAVE BEEN IMMERSED in learning about the concepts of vibrational energy for the past 15 years. The best book I have ever seen on the subject of vibrational and energy medicine is Richard Gerber's groundbreaking book *Vibrational Medicine*, which was released in 1986. I understand from other spiritual healers that Gerber wrote the book when he was 33 years old. I cannot believe that a mortal human being could write such a profound and breathtaking book at such a young age.

Spiritual healers have told me that this information was channeled to Gerber from angelic intervention. Even though this book is approximately 30 years old, I believe the information still is authentic and valid. Gerber was decades ahead of his time and perhaps one of the earliest messengers revealing the astounding information regarding energetic and vibrational medicine. Gerber inspired me and motivated me to dig deeper into myself in order to understand the nature of vibration. Through his inspiration, I have lectured all over the world on metabolic and vibrational medicine.

My most recent lecture, "Good Vibes versus Bad," discusses the essence of why some vibrations can be harmful, while others are healing for the body. I have combined nuggets of insight from that lecture here. I share them with you in hopes that you consider the message as important as I have, since maintaining a high vibration will keep you healthy, happy, and whole, while a low vibration does the opposite.

Let me start with a list of behaviors, activities, and attitudes that will affect your vibration negatively. Check yourself against this list to see if you are harboring any feelings, emotions, or thoughts or doing any regular activities that may be keeping your personal vibration artificially low. Your energetic vibration may not be at its natural level because it is being suppressed by thoughts or actions not conducive to high vibrational energy. Consider which items on this list you can correct.

- Thinking negatively, pessimistically

- Lacking love

- Lacking faith

- Being fearful

- Lacking spiritual connections

- Lacking emotional connections

- Having aggressive behavior

- Being selfish

- Remaining isolated and being lonely

- Feeling judged or rejected

- Lacking a support system

- Lacking a purpose

- Having envy

- Being greedy

- Having ego

- Leaving sadness or grief unresolved

- Staying angry

- Lacking compassion

- Lacking forgiveness of self or others

- Lacking flexibility

- Lacking a creative outlet for expression

- Being cruel or experiencing cruelty by others

- Losing a job

- Lacking activity and physical movement

- Being unable to recognize your blessings

- Eating a poor diet

- Being lazy

- Using drugs

- Drinking alcohol

- Consuming excess sugars

- Eating GMO (genetically modified organism) foods

- Overexposing yourself to the chaotic, unseen frequencies of cordless and cellular phones, Bluetooth monitors, cell phone towers, computers, and other wireless technologies that create the invisible toxicity surrounding the Earth

We must all work to avoid the trap of living in a "false self." Tell the truth. Any misrepresentation of the truth, or falsehood, is a betrayal of the self. Nothing will bring your vibration down faster than if your life is a lie, you fail to pursue an authentic existence, or you just don't tell the truth!

Now, here is a list of behaviors, activities, and attitudes that will raise your vibration.

- Having faith

- Loving yourself and others

- Forgiving yourself and others

- Counting your blessings; being grateful

- Being compassionate

- Having empathy for others

- Seeking joy and happiness

- Maintaining healthy emotional and strong spiritual connections

- Creating and maintaining friendships

- Creating biological and spiritual family connections and building romantic relationships

- Letting go of anger, fear, ego, grief, and selfishness

- Being flexible and fluid

- Spending time with children and animals

- Spending time in nature

- Giving to charity

- Praying

- Being in service to others

- Reducing stressful situations

- Being a positive thinker

- Eating a clean, non-GMO, organic foods–based diet

- Exercising

- Practicing meditation

- Including self-care rituals such as yoga and massage

- Not using illegal drugs

- Limiting alcohol intake

- Volunteering

- Being creative

- Using your imagination

- Pursuing a favorite hobby

- Watching inspirational films

- Paying attention and giving compliments

- Listening to music

- Singing and/or dancing

- Smiling and laughing a lot

- Grounding to the Earth in your bare feet

- Taking targeted nutritional supplements that support Vital Force energy

- Drinking clean water with minerals, preferably out of glass containers

This list is by no means comprehensive. With a little thought and ingenuity, you can probably add to this list or create your own. The key is to connect as fully as possible with who you are and what makes you happy. When you are in a state of happiness and bliss, your vibration will be at its highest. If you're not sure how to achieve that, try to be still and listen for answers or direction. Meditate or pray and ask for guidance from the ascendant masters. Frequently, in a flash—as fleeting as a thief in the night—the message will be revealed in your intuition. Listen carefully because the insight represents universal truth.

Our human connection is undeniable. We can think differently, act differently, make vastly different choices, and have wildly different ideals, but in the end, we humans are fundamentally the same. That is the underlying message in the health revelations given to a simple man who had a powerful near-death experience and returned with life-changing information that is true for every human being on the planet. The interconnectedness of all things is real and pure and the spiritual consciousness of the planet is definitely increasing. The number of near-death experiencers coming forward reflects benevolent unseen energies, which is a testimony of light from the spiritual realm. Tommy and other NDErs are the canaries in the coal mine— or messengers to all mankind. In the final analysis, we should be asking ourselves the most important questions, such as:

Why am I here?

What is my life's true purpose?

When and how do I prepare for going home?

Blessings,
Dr. Stephen Sinatra

ACKNOWLEDGMENTS

IT IS WITH DEEP gratitude and appreciation that we acknowledge the following individuals who brought the Sinatras and the Rosas together in the spirit of connection.

Our trail of connectedness begins with Rick and Melody Spano, who first suggested to Tommy Rosa that it was time to tell his heavenly story and that it would make a great book.

To Joe Bucci, a dear friend to Tommy and a true believer.

To Susan Johnson, who first introduced Tommy to Dr. Sinatra's life-changing and lifesaving book, *Metabolic Cardiology*, during his health crisis and talked about Dr. Stephen Sinatra, who lived near her and was known to think "outside the box."

To Dr. Richard and Cindy Becker, who host the television show *Your Health*, which featured Dr. Sinatra. Tommy first saw Dr. Sinatra, his heart hero, and received his healing messages while watching their program.

To Donna LeClare, who encouraged Tommy, despite his physical health challenges at the time, to attend a health conference in Saint Petersburg, Florida, where he and Dr. Sinatra met in person for the first time.

And to Dr. Lee Cowden, a deeply spiritual man who regularly brings the best of all worlds together and holds the greatest integrative conferences. Dr. Cowden gave Dr. Sinatra and Tommy Rosa the opportunity to address his conference attendees and introduce their amazing story.

As the idea for the book evolved from concept to reality, our connection continues with Dr. Ibrahim Karim, who gave us encouragement and knowledge.

To Dr. J. J. and Desiree Hurtak, who also provided inspiration and clarity.

To Lindi Stoler, who grasped the spiritual importance of the story and helped shape the early direction of the project. Lindi introduced us to Steve Troha, our literary agent and now a treasured friend who took interest and leadership in the project from the day he received it. Steve has been there for us every step of the way. We owe a huge debt to Steve for all he has done and continues to do to get the book and its messages of health, healing, and well-being out into the world.

To Maggie Greenwood-Robinson, our brilliant collaborator, who figured out how to blend the divine revelations from Heaven with the wisdom of Earth.

To JoAnne Piazza, Dr. Sinatra's tireless and dedicated executive assistant, who spent endless hours at the computer during the final editing process.

And to editorial director Jennifer Levesque and the rest of the Rodale team, Mary Ann Naples, Gail Gonzales, Leah Miller, Kristin Kiser, Yelena Nesbit, Brent Gallenberger, Emily Weber Eagen, Susan Turner, Melissa Olund, Chris De Marchis, Jean Lee, and Mollie Thomas. This team has encouraged and supported the publication of this book, and to them we owe the deepest gratitude.

And to all of our wonderful endorsers with whom we are deeply connected and who each took the time to review the manuscript. Despite their various faiths and belief systems, our endorsers recognized the universal value inherent in the divine guidance and earthly direction on how to heal the mind, body, and spirit. They include Dr. Christiane Northrup, physician, leading authority in women's health and wellness, and author of *Goddesses Never Age*; Dannion Brinkley, near-death experiencer and author; Dr. Joe Mercola, osteopathic physician, alternative medicine proponent, Web entrepreneur, and author; Dr. Nicholas Perricone, board-certified clinical and research dermatologist and author; Suzanne Somers, actress, entrepreneur, and author; Dr. Bernie Siegel, physician, surgeon, and author; JJ Virgin, fitness and nutrition expert and author; Dr. Robert Thurman, professor, Buddhist scholar, and author; Eva Herr, radio show host, alternative holistic counselor, and author; Dr. Larry Dossey, physician, leader in alternative medicine and spirituality, and author; Dr. Mark Hyman, physician, author, founder, and medical director of the UltraWellness Center; Dr. Richard and Cindy Becker, cohosts of the TV show *Your Health* and authors; Dr. David Perlmutter, physician, author, and president of the Perlmutter Health Center; and Dr. Nathan Katz, distinguished professor and author.

And finally, to our deepest, most beloved connections, Jan Sinatra and Michelle Christopher Rosa. This book has undergone a five-year evolution. Our heartfelt gratitude to our wives and soul mates, who shared our vision of bringing Tommy's story into the world. In addition to their full emotional support, they worked long and tirelessly on the many versions of this book as it evolved into *Health Revelations from Heaven.*

BIBLIOGRAPHY

Aron, A., et al. 2005. Reward, motivation, and emotion systems associated with early-stage intense romantic love. *Journal of Neurophysiology* 94:327–37.

Bodicoat, D. H., et al. 2015. Is the number of fast-food outlets in the neighbourhood related to screen-detected type 2 diabetes mellitus and associated risk factors? *Public Health Nutrition* 18:1698–1705.

Carson, J. W., et al. 2005. Forgiveness and chronic low back pain: a preliminary study examining the relationship of forgiveness to pain, anger, and psychological stress. *Journal of Pain* 6:84–91.

Chevalier, G., et al. 2012. Earthing: health implications of reconnecting the human body to the Earth's surface electrons. *Journal of Environmental and Public Health* 2012:291541.

Chevalier, G. 2015. The effect of grounding the human body on mood. *Psychology Reports* 116:534–43.

Childs, E., et al. 2014. Personality traits modulate emotional and physiological responses to stress. *Behavioural Pharmacology* 25:493–502.

Danner, D. D., et al. 2001. Positive emotions in early life and longevity: findings from the nun study. *Journal of Personality and Social Psychology* 80:804–13.

Davis, D. L., et al. 2013. Swedish review strengthens grounds for concluding that radiation from cellular and cordless phones is a probable human carcinogen. *Pathophysiology* 20:123–29.

De Felice, F. G., and Ferreira, S. T. 2014. Inflammation, defective insulin signaling, and mitochondrial dysfunction as common molecular denominators connecting type 2 diabetes to Alzheimer's disease. *Diabetes* 63:2262–72.

Editor. 2011. Scientists probe brushes with the afterlife. State News Service, February 11.

Emoto, M. 2004. Healing with water. *Journal of Alternative and Complementary Medicine* 10:19–21.

Engel, G. L. 1975. The death of a twin: mourning and anniversary reactions. Fragments of 10 years of self-analysis. *The International Journal of Psycho-Analysis* 56:23–40.

Friedmann, E., and Thomas, S. A. 1995. Pet ownership, social support, and one-year survival after acute myocardial infarction in the Cardiac Arrhythmia Suppression Trial (CAST). *American Journal of Cardiology* 76:1213–17.

Gaby, A. R. 2010. Nutritional treatments for acute myocardial infarction. *Alternative Medicine Review* July; 15(2):113–23.

Gerber, R. 1986. *Vibrational Medicine,* Rochester, Vermont: Bear & Company.

Havas, M. 2013. Radiation from wireless technology affects the blood, the heart, and the autonomic nervous system. *Reviews on Environmental Health* 28:75–84.

Hawkley, L. C., and Cacioppo, J. T. 2003. Loneliness and pathways to disease. *Brain, Behavior, and Immunity* Supplement 1:S98–105.

Jamieson, K., et al. 2007. The effects of electric fields on charged molecules and particles in individual microenvironments. *Atmospheric Environment* 41: 5224–35.

King, M. S., et al. 2002. Transcendental meditation, hypertension and heart disease. *Australian Family Physician* 31:164–68.

Klotter, J. 2002. Vibrational frequencies that heal. *Townsend Letter for Doctors and Patients,* May 1.

Kong, Y., et al. 2014. Oxidative stress, mitochondrial dysfunction, and the mitochondria theory of aging. *Interdisciplinary Topics in Gerontology* 39:86–107.

Kubzansky, L. D., et al. 2001. Is the glass half empty or half full? A prospective study of optimism and coronary heart disease in the normative aging study. *Psychosomatic Medicine* 63:910–16.

Maxwell, J. 2010. The "big 5" challenges people face: don't let your attitude set you back. *Success,* September 1.

Mincolla, M. 2013. *Whole Health.* New York: Jeremy Tarcher, pp. 19–20.

Mooventhan, A., and Khode, V. 2014. Effect of Bhramari pranayama and OM chanting on pulmonary function in healthy individuals: a prospective randomized control trial. *International Journal of Yoga* 7:104–10.

Naughton, A. M., et al. 2013. Emotional, behavioral, and developmental features indicative of neglect or emotional abuse in preschool children: a systematic review. *Journal of the American Medical Association—Pediatrics* 167:769–75.

Newton, T., et al. 2008. Lack of a close confidant: prevalence and correlates in a medically underserved primary care sample. *Psychology, Health & Medicine* 13:185–92.

Nidich, S. I., et al. 2009. A randomized controlled trial on effects of the Transcendental Meditation program on blood pressure, psychological distress, and coping in young adults. *American Journal of Hypertension* 22:1326–31.

Nogueira, C., et al. 2014. Syndromes associated with mitochondrial DNA depletion. *Italian Journal of Pediatrics* 40:34.

Okereke, O. I., et al. 2012. High phobic anxiety is related to lower leukocyte telomere length in women. *PLoS One* 7:e40516.

Oschman, J., et al. 2015. The effects of grounding (earthing) on inflammation, the immune response, wound healing, and prevention of chronic inflammatory and autoimmune diseases. *Journal of Inflammation Research* 8:83–96.

Oshita, D., et al. 2013. A Buddhist-based meditation practice for care and healing: an introduction and its application. *International Journal of Nursing Practice* 19:15–23.

Pauly, D. F., and Pepine, C. J. 2000. D-ribose as a supplement for cardiac energy metabolism. *Journal of Cardiovascular Pharmacology and Therapeutics* 5:249–58.

Ranheim, P. 2008. Editor. Chemical Sensitivity. American Academy of Environmental Medicine, AAEMonline.org.

Robards, J., et al. 2012. Marital status, health and mortality. *Maturitas* 73:295–99.

Robles, T. F., and Kiecolt-Glaser, J. K. 2003. The physiology of marriage: pathways to health. *Physiology & Behavior* 79:409–16.

Schachter-Shalomi, Z. 1995. *From Age-Ing to Sage-Ing: A Revolutionary Approach to Growing Older.* New York: Warner Books.

Sinatra, D. 2015. Naturopathic Medicine and the Prevention and Treatment of Cardiovascular Disease. In *Nutritional and Integrative Strategies in Cardiovascular Medicine,* ed. S. T. Sinatra and M. Houston, 179–204. Boca Raton, Florida: CRC Press.

Sinatra, S. T. 2011. Earthing update—outstanding benefits . . . with a few caveats. *Townsend Letter,* May 1.

Sinatra, S. T. 2011. *The Sinatra Solution/Metabolic Cardiology.* Basic Health Publications, Laguna Beach, CA.

Sinatra, S. T. 2009. Metabolic cardiology: the missing link in cardiovascular disease. *Alternative Therapies in Health and Medicine* 15:48–50.

Sinatra, S. T., Roberts, J. C., and Zucker M. 2007. *Reverse Heart Disease Now: Stop Deadly Cardiovascular Plaque Before It's Too Late.* John Wiley & Sons, Inc., Hoboken, NJ.

Solanki, M. S., et al. 2013. Music as a therapy: role in psychiatry. *Asian Journal of Psychiatry* 6:193–99.

Tang, H. Y., and Vezeau, T. 2003. The use of music intervention in healthcare research: a narrative review of the literature. *Journal of Nursing Research* 18:174–90.

van Lommel, P., et al. 2001. Near-death experience in survivors of cardiac arrest: a prospective study in the Netherlands. *The Lancet* 358:2039–45.

Williams, R. B., et al. 1992. Prognostic importance of social and economic resources among medically treated patients with angiographically documented coronary artery disease. *Journal of the American Medical Association* 267:520–24.

Yang, Q., et al. 2014. Added sugar intake and cardiovascular diseases mortality among U.S. adults. *JAMA Internal Medicine* 174:516–24.

INDEX

Underscored references indicate charts.

Printed in the United States
by Baker & Taylor Publisher Services